THE PA BIBLE

A PANCE Workbook Written by the Physician Assistants Who Wish They'd Had It

PART 2

Christine Nelson,
Tiffany Lee,
&
Meredith Allen

The PA Bible: A PANCE Workbook Written by the Physician Assistants Who Wish They'd Had It

PART 2

NELSON, CHRISTINE, Author
THE PA BIBLE
CHRISTINE NELSON

In Association with:
ELITE ONLINE PUBLISHING
63 East 11400 South #230
Sandy, UT 84070
EliteOnlinePublishing.com

ISBN: 978-1-971310-06-0 (Paperback)
MED058210
MED086000

Why We Created This Workbook

Our hope is that PA students can have most everything needed to study for the PANCE in one place, this workbook. While studying for the PANCE ourselves we spent hundreds of dollars on different books and online systems and felt overwhelmed by the options and at times too much information. We wanted to create a workbook that was directly tailored to the PANCE blueprint, user-friendly, and concise enough as to not be overwhelming. This workbook is specifically designed to categorize necessary information while allowing the student to participate in the process by filling in the information, which has been proven to help with recall and retention.

How to Use This Workbook

- We recognize some of the topics fit into multiple subjects, but we kept it simple by only putting each topic in one place in the workbook. You can find each topic in the appendix if it isn't where you instinctively think it would be.
- Some topics may not have enough room to put everything in that you learn. We recommend putting in the information that is harder to remember, and not writing what you already know. This will help to ensure that your individual workbook doesn't become overcrowded or busy.
- There are "empty" boxes within the workbook that are intended for the reader to draw or fill in that information, again this helps with recollection and learning.
- There is a section at the end of each chapter to put the most commonly used medications within each subject.
- There are also lined pages at the end of each subject so that you can add any subjects or information that you feel are important but that aren't specifically on the PANCE blueprint.

Table of Contents

Infectious Disease

Viral Diseases

Herpes Simplex Virus 1: "Cold sore"

Sx: Tingling sensation (prodrome), vesicles can cross vermillion border

PE:

Dx:

Tx:

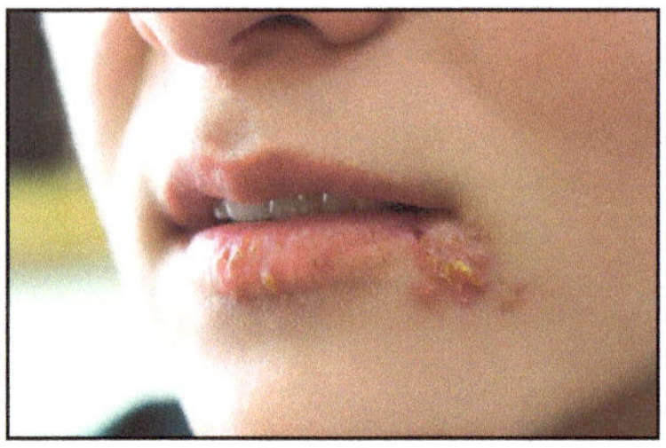

Herpes Simplex Virus 2: Genital lesions/ulcers

Sx: Painful ulcers and/or vesicular lesions that progress to ulcerations

PE:

Dx:

Tx:

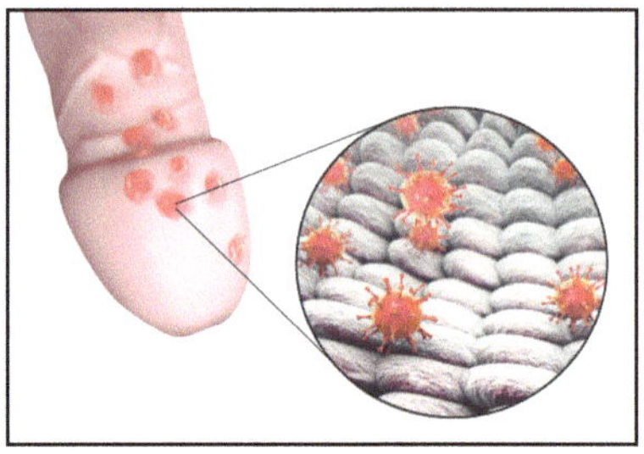

Herpes Simplex Virus 3 (Varicella Zoster "VZV" or "Shingles"):

Sx:

PE:

Dx: Clinical, Tzanck smear, polymerase chain reaction (PCR)

Tx:

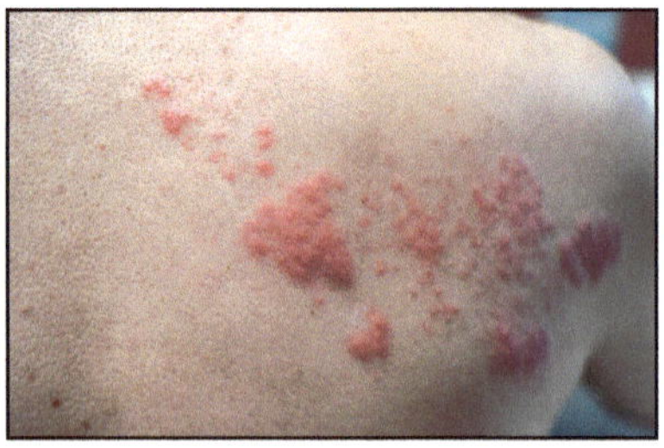

Herpes Simplex Virus 4 (Epstein-Barr virus "EBV"): Mononucleosis

Complications:

Sx: Fever + posterior cervical lymphadenopathy + pharyngitis, splenomegaly

PE:

Dx:

Tx:

Herpes Simplex Virus (Cytomegalovirus "CMV"): Mononucleosis

Sx: Malaise, fever, N/V/D

PE:

Dx:

Tx:

Herpes Simplex Virus 6 & 7 (Roseola "6th disease"):

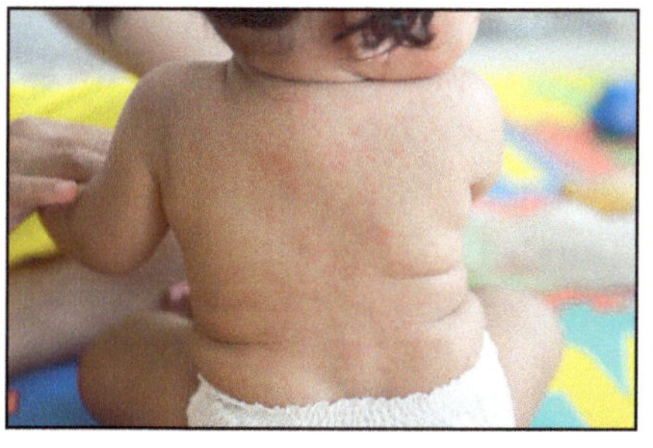

Sx: Fever, exanthem rash

PE:

Dx:

Tx:

Herpes Simplex Virus 8 (Kaposi Sarcoma): AIDS related

Sx: Skin lesion (purple), oral lesion, LAD, weight loss

PE:

Dx:

Tx:

Human Immunodeficiency Virus (HIV): Retrovirus

AIDS: CD4 < 200 w/opportunistic infection

Sx: Fever, night sweats, weight loss, skin rashes, oral ulcers

PE:

Dx: ELISA (sensitive), Western blot (specific)

Tx:

Human Papillomavirus (HPV): Linked to cervical & oropharyngeal cancers

Types: Cutaneous warts (1,2,4), genital warts (6, 11), cancerous (16, 18)

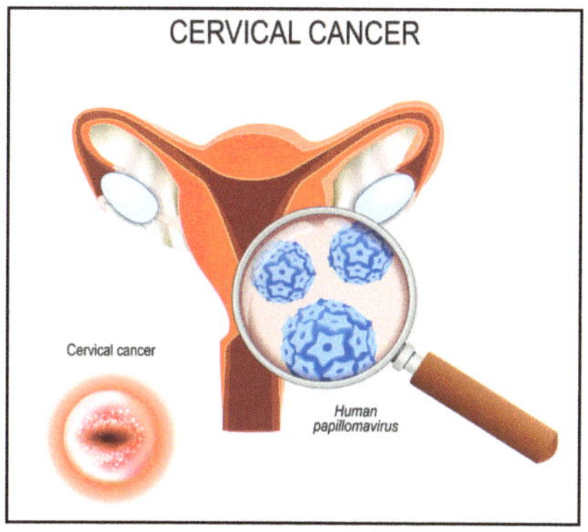

Sx:

PE:

Dx: Biopsy, PAP smear

Tx:

Mumps: Paramyxovirus

Complications: Orchitis, aseptic meningitis, pancreatitis

Sx:

PE:

Dx: Elevated amylase, leukopenia, + IgM and IgG.

______________________________________ Tx:

____

____

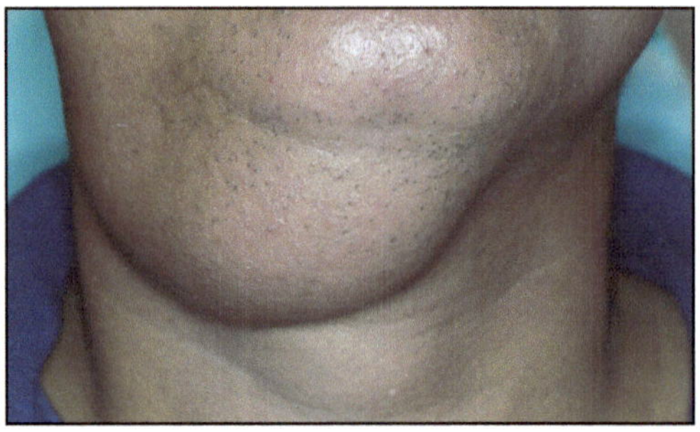

Rabies: CNS infection

Transmission: Via animals including unvaccinated house pets (dogs)

Sx:

PE:

Dx: Gram stain negri bodies, polymerase chain reaction (PCR)

______________________________________ Tx:

____

____

Parasitic Diseases

Amebiasis (Entamoeba Histolytica): Protozoa

Sx:

PE:

Dx: Stool antigen, serum antibody

Tx:

Malaria: Protozoa

Protective Factors: Sickle cell trait and thalassemia trait

Sx: Cyclical fever (3 days), anemia, coma

PE:

Dx: Giemsa stain smear

Tx:

Babesiosis: Protozoa
Transmission: Ticks

Sx: Fever, hemolytic anemia, jaundice

PE:

Dx:

Tx:

Toxoplasmosis: Protozoa

Transmission: Cat feces & raw pork

Congenital: Blueberry muffin rash

Sx:

PE:

Dx: Anti-Toxoplasma IgG (serum) & IgM (serum)

Tx:

Chagas Disease (American Trypanosomiasis): Trypanosoma cruzi (T. cruzi)

Sx: Acute-

Latent-

PE:

Dx: CBC, microscopy

Tx:

Trichinellosis: Roundworm

Transmission: Consumption of raw pork

Sx: Periorbital/facial edema, myositis, fever

PE:

Dx:

Tx:

Ascariasis: Roundworm

Transmission: Poor sanitation, travel to endemic areas

Sx:

PE:

Dx: Stool microscopy, chest or abdominal X-ray

Tx:

Enterobius (Pinworms):

Transmission: Fecal-oral, thumb sucking

Sx: Perianal itching (worse at night) & perianal erythema

PE:

Dx: Scotch tape test

Tx:

Cestodes (Tapeworms):

Sx: GI symptoms, weight loss, seizures, hepatomegaly

PE:

Dx:

Tx:

Hookworms:

Transmission: Enter through feet from infected soil, goes into lungs, gets coughed up then swallowed into gastrointestinal tract

Sx:

PE:

Dx: Clinical = skin scrapings/biopsy, eggs in feces

Tx:

Leishmaniasis: Sandfly bite (protozoa)

Sx: Cutaneous ulcers, visceral hepatosplenomegaly, fever

PE:

Dx: CBC, LFT's, BUN, hCG

Tx:

Fungal Diseases

Candidiasis:

Sx: Esophagitis, oral thrush, vaginal, fungemia, endocarditis

PE:

Dx: KOH with budding yeast and pseudohyphae

Tx:

Cryptococcosis: Most common in patients with HIV infection and immunosuppression

Transmission: Pigeon droppings

Sx: Meningitis, pneumonia, constitutional symptoms

PE:

Dx:

Tx:

Histoplasmosis: Michigan & Ohio River Valley, most common in patients with AIDS

Transmission: Bat and bird droppings

Sx: Fever, headache, non-productive cough, pleuritic chest pain

PE:

Dx:

Tx:

Pneumocystis: P. jirovecii, most common in patients with AIDS (CD4 cell count < 200 cells/microliter)

Sx:

PE:

Dx: Chest X-ray with bilateral peri-hilar infiltrates, high LDH

Tx:

Aspergillosis:

Sx:

PE:

Dx: Chest X-ray, high-resolution chest CT scan, MRI of brain & sinuses

Tx:

Mucormycosis:

Sx: Sinus and facial pain, proptosis, skin nodules, black eschars

PE:

Dx:

Tx:

Coccidioidomycosis: "Valley fever", southwestern USA

Sx:

PE:

Dx: Sputum culture, enzyme immunoassay serology

Tx:

Blastomycosis: Pulmonary, cutaneous, disseminated

Sx: Fever, weight loss, fatigue, cough, skin lesion

PE:

Dx:

Tx:

Bacterial Respiratory Diseases

Diphtheria: **Corynebacterium diphtheria (gram-positive rod)**

Sx: Sore throat, pseudo membrane formation, neck swelling

PE:

Dx:

Tx:

Mycobacterium Avium Complex: **Prior lung disease, most common in patients with AIDS**

Sx:

PE:

Dx: CBC, LFT, sputum culture (acid fast), X-ray

Tx:

Other Bacterial Diseases

Methicillin-Resistant Staphylococcus Aureus (MRSA): S. aureus resistant to methicillin (usually various other drugs) most common in immunocompromised patients or IV drug users

Sx: Skin lesions - pustules on an erythematous base, gold/salmon sputum

PE:

Dx:

Tx:

Rocky Mountain Spotted Fever: Rickettsia ricketsii (gram-negative, obligate intracellular)
Transmission: Ticks

Sx: Centripetal rash (outside in), fever, rash, headache

PE:

Dx:

Tx:

Erythema Migrans (Lyme Disease): Borrelia burgdorferi (gram-negative spirochete)
Transmission: Deer tick

Sx: Bull's eye rash, cardiac arrythmias, chronic arthritis
Early disease vs. late disease

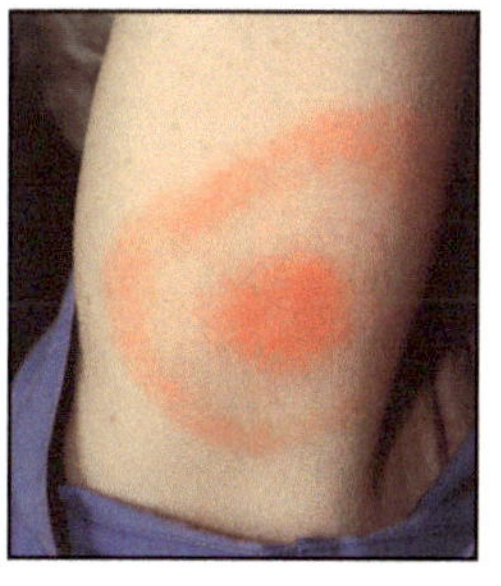

PE:

Dx:

Tx:

Zika: Transmitted by mosquitos
Dangerous in pregnancy

Sx:

PE:

Dx: Reverse transcriptase-polymerase chain reaction (RT-PCR), serology

Tx:

Cat Scratch: Bartonella henselae (gram-negative coccobacillli)

Sx: Ulcer, fever, lymphadenopathy, papular or pustular lesion

PE:

Dx: Serology, culture

Tx:

Tularemia: Gram-negative coccobacillli
Transmission: Tick, biting fly, rabbits, and other infected animals

Sx:

PE:

Dx: Serology, blood and specimen culture, PCR of ulcer or lymph

Tx:

Brucellosis: Gram-negative coccobacilli

Transmission: Infected animal products, usually milk or cheese

Sx: Fever, chills, constitutional symptoms, arthralgias

PE:

Dx:

Tx:

Plague: Yersinia pestis (gram-negative rod)

Sx: Bubonic:

Yersiniosis:

Pneumonic:

Dx: Bubonic:

Pneumonic:

Yersiniosis:

Tx:

Necrotizing Fasciitis:

Sx: Bullae, gangrene, fever, nausea, vomiting

PE:

Dx:

Tx:

Bacterial STIs

Chlamydia: Obligate intracellular gram-negative rod

Sx: White discharge or asymptomatic, white cervical or penile discharge, friable cervix

PE: Post-coital bleeding (female)

Dx:

Tx:

Gonorrhea: Neisseria gonorrhoeae (gram-negative diplococci)

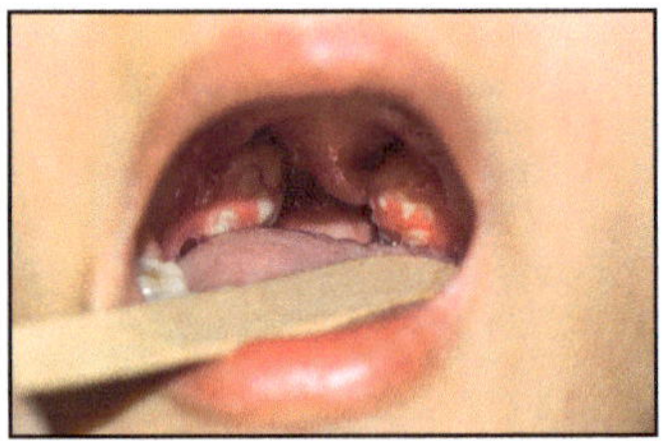

Sx: Asymptomatic OR yellow, purulent discharge,
urethritis, cervicitis, epididymitis, prostatitis,
risk of pelvic inflammatory disease (PID) in women

PE:

Dx:

Tx:

Syphilis: Treponema pallidum (spirochete)

Sx: 1. Primary:
2. Secondary:
3. Tertiary:

Congenital - Hutchinson teeth, saddle-nose deformity, keratitis

Dx: Darkfield microscopy of chancre
Sensitive:
Specific:

Tx:

Chancroid: **Haemophilus ducreyi (gram-negative coccobacillus)**

Sx: Painful genital ulcers, inguinal lymphadenopathy

PE:

Dx:

Tx:

Lymphogranuloma Venereum (LGV):

Sx: Inguinal lymphadenopathy, fever, malaise, arthralgias, lower abdominal or lower back pain

Stage 1:

Stage 2:

Stage 3:

PE:

Dx: NAAT (genital or lymph node specimens)

Tx:

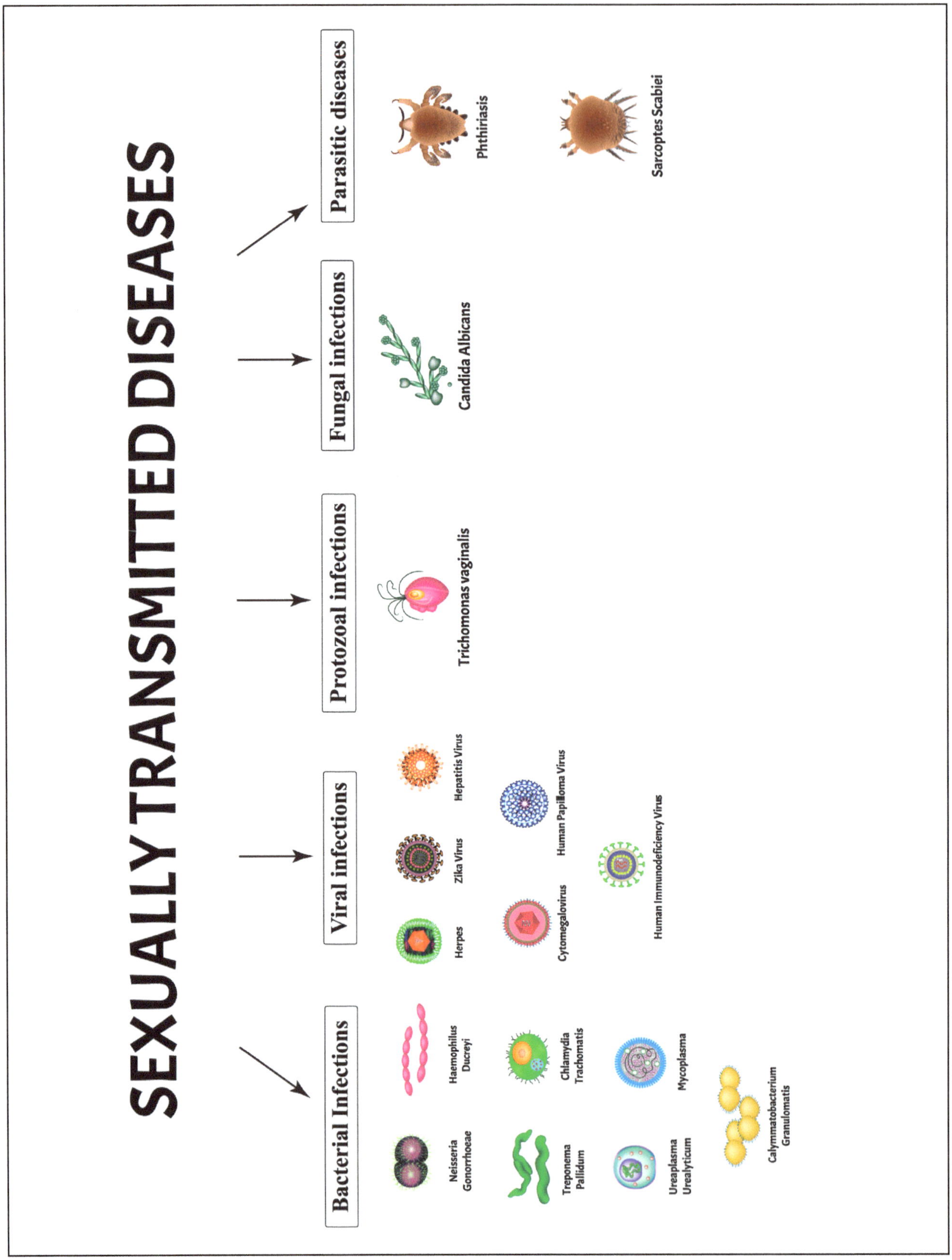
SEXUALLY TRANSMITTED DISEASES
Bacterial Infections
Neisseria Gonorrhoeae
Haemophilus Ducreyi
Treponema Pallidum
Chlamydia Trachomatis
Ureaplasma Urealyticum
Mycoplasma
Calymmatobacterium Granulomatis
Viral infections
Herpes
Zika Virus
Hepatitis Virus
Cytomegalovirus
Human Papilloma Virus
Human Immunodeficiency Virus
Protozoal infections
Trichomonas vaginalis
Fungal infections
Candida Albicans
Parasitic diseases
Phthiriasis
Sarcoptes Scabiei

Bacterial Gastrointestinal Diseases

Campylobacter Jejuni: **Gram-negative curved rod**

Transmission: Contaminated meat or milk

Sx: Abdominal pain, diarrhea, headache, myalgias, chills, fever

PE:

Dx:

Tx:

Botulism: **Clostridium botulinum (gram-positive, anaerobic rod with spores)**

Transmission:

Sx: Flaccid paralysis, respiratory distress, "floppy baby" syndrome

PE:

Dx:

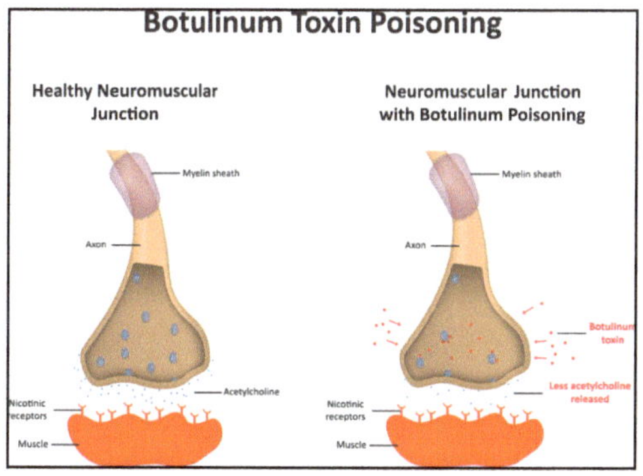

Tx:

Anthrax: **Gram-positive rod with spores**

Sx:

PE:

Dx:

Tx:

Bacterial Neurologic Diseases

Tetanus: Gram-positive, anaerobic rod, neurotoxin

Sx: Trismus (lock jaw), back pain, dysphagia, muscle spasms

PE:

Dx:

________________________________ Tx:

____

____

Meningococcal Meningitis: Neisseria meningitides (gram-negative diploccoci)

Sx: Nuchal rigidity + fever + HA, purpuric rash

(+) Kernig's:

(+) Brudzinski's:

PE:

Dx:

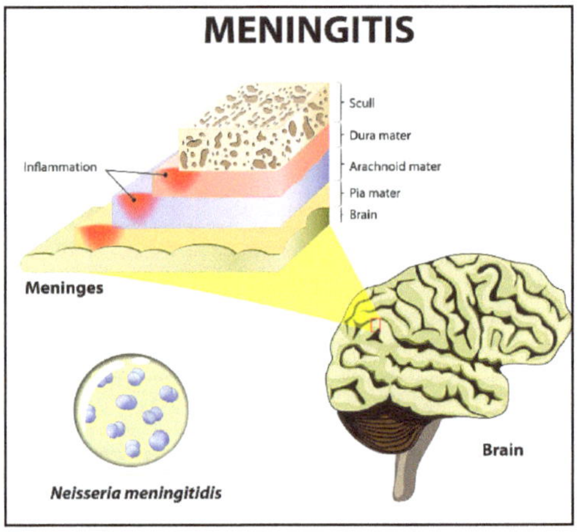

____

____

____

Tx:

Listeriosis: Gram-positive rod

Common causes: Exposure to contaminated food

Sx:

PE:

Dx: CBC, brain MRI & CT

________________________________ Tx:

____

____

Vaginal Infections

Candida Vaginitis:

Sx: Thick, curdy, white discharge

PE:

Dx: Wet mount = pseudo hyphae "spaghetti & meatballs"

____

____

____

Tx:

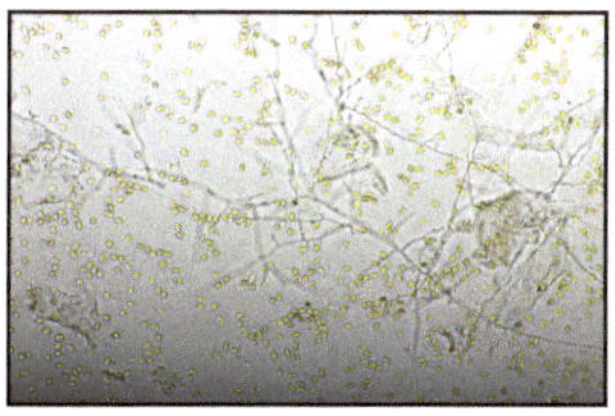

Bacterial Vaginosis:

Sx: Thin, white/grey discharge

PE:

Dx: Wet mount = clue cells

____

____

____

Tx:

Trichomoniasis:

Sx: Frothy, green/yellow discharge

PE:

Dx: Wet mount = motile trichomonads

____

____

____

Tx:

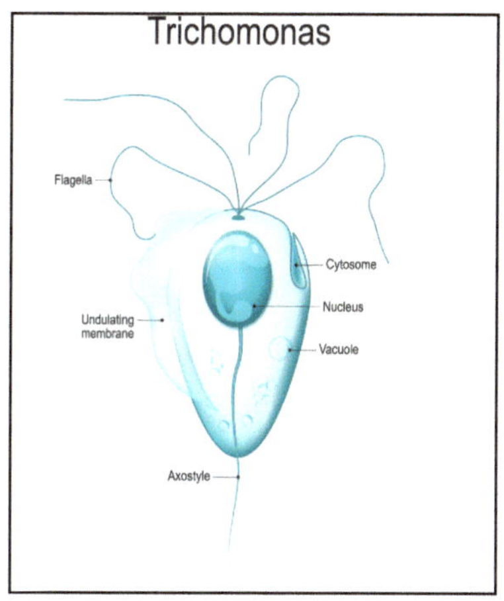

Pelvic Inflammatory Disease (PID):

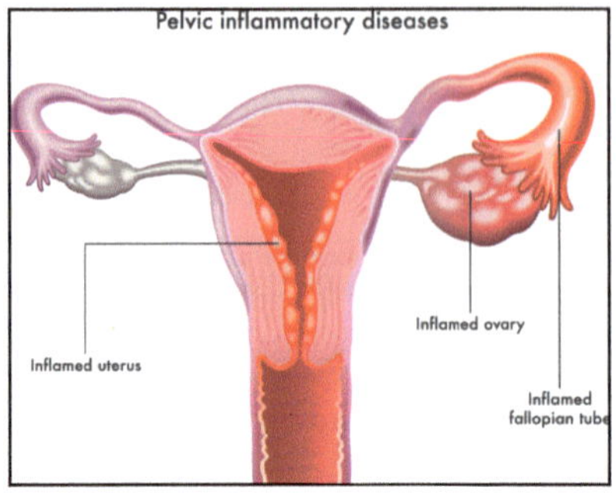

Sx:

PE: Chandelier sign (cervical motion tenderness), adnexal mass

Dx: Labs = high WBC > 10,000, fever

____

____

____

Tx:

Tubo-Ovarian Abscess: Usually follows PID

Sx:

Dx: Pelvic US

____

____

____

Tx:

Mycoplasma Pneumoniae: In Pulm

Pertussis "Whooping Cough": In Pulm

Tuberculosis: In Pulm

Rheumatic Fever: In Cardio

Cholera: In GI

Pharyngitis (Strep Throat): In EENT

Pityriasis Rosea: In Derm

Haemophilus Influenzae: In Pulm

Salmonella: In GI

Shigella: In GI

Condyloma Acuminatum: In Derm

Medications

____________: MOA = ____________
Indication(s)= ____________
Side Effects = ____________
Types/ Examples = ____________

____

____

____________: MOA = ____________
Indication(s)= ____________
Side Effects = ____________
Types/ Examples = ____________

____

____

____________: MOA = ____________
Indication(s)= ____________
Side Effects = ____________
Types/ Examples = ____________

____

____

____________: MOA = ____________
Indication(s)= ____________
Side Effects = ____________
Types/ Examples = ____________

____

____

____________: MOA = ____________
Indication(s)= ____________
Side Effects = ____________
Types/ Examples = ____________

____

____

Medications

____________________: **MOA =** ____

Indication(s)=____

Side Effects = ____

Types/ Examples = ____

____________________: **MOA =** ____

Indication(s)=____

Side Effects = ____

Types/ Examples = ____

____________________: **MOA =** ____

Indication(s)=____

Side Effects = ____

Types/ Examples = ____

____________________: **MOA =** ____

Indication(s)=____

Side Effects = ____

Types/ Examples = ____

____________________: **MOA =** ____

Indication(s)=____

Side Effects = ____

Types/ Examples = ____

Dermatology

Atopic Dermatitis (Eczema):

Sx: Asthma, allergic rhinitis, pruritis, erythema, scaling, vesicles, papules
FLEXOR SURFACES

PE:

Dx:

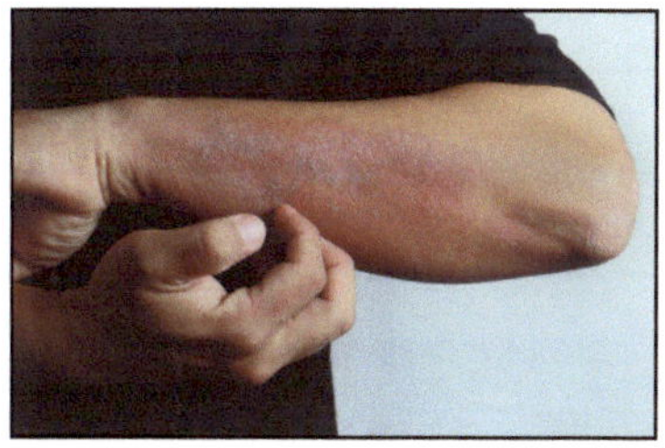

____

____

____

Tx:

Dyshidrotic Eczema:

Sx: Tapioca-like bumps, itchy, symmetric

PE:

Dx:

____

____

____

Tx:

Psoriasis:

Sx: Hyperpigmented, thick, leathery, sharp margins, silvery scales
Extensor surfaces

PE:

Dx: KOBNER phenomenon - AUSPITZ sign

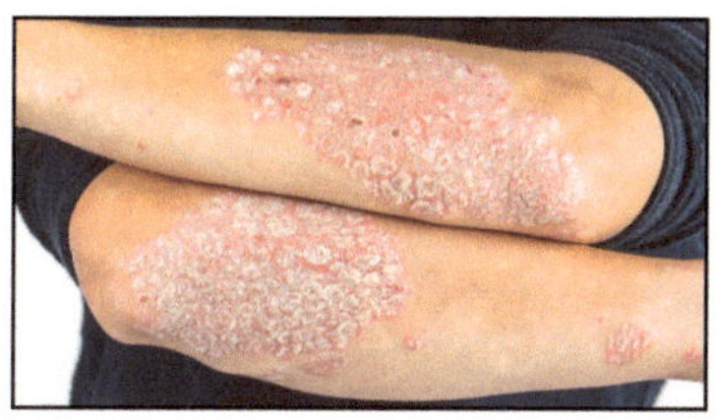

____

____

____

Tx:

Lichen Planus:

Sx: Itchy, flat-topped bumps,

PE: Purple, Papule, Polygonal, Pruritis, Planar

Dx: KOEBNER phenomenon

Wickham's Striae (white lines)

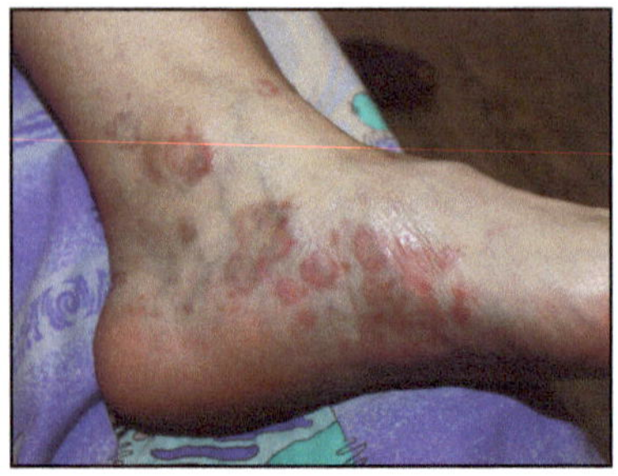

Tx:

Lichen Simplex Chronicus: Atopic dermatitis is precursor

Sx: Lichenified plaques & excoriations, doesn't bleed when scratched

PE:

Dx:

Tx:

Urticaria:

Sx: Allergic reaction - blanchable, pruritic, raised, erythematous or skin-colored papules, wheels or plaques on skin

PE: Darier's sign

Dx:

Tx:

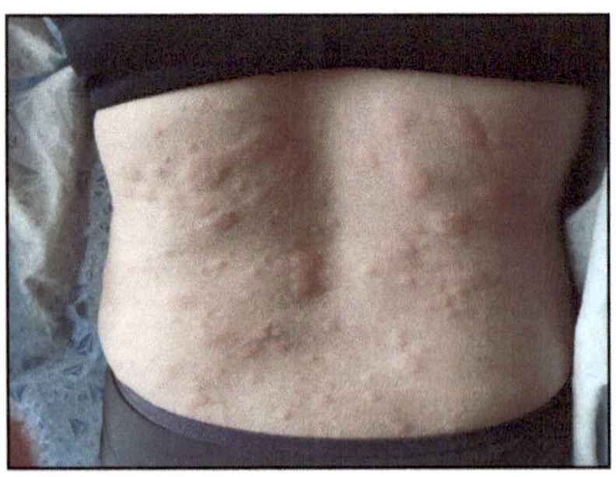

Diaper Dermatitis/Candida & Fungal Infection: **Irritant contact dermatitis**

Sx:

PE:

Dx:

____________________ Tx:

____

____

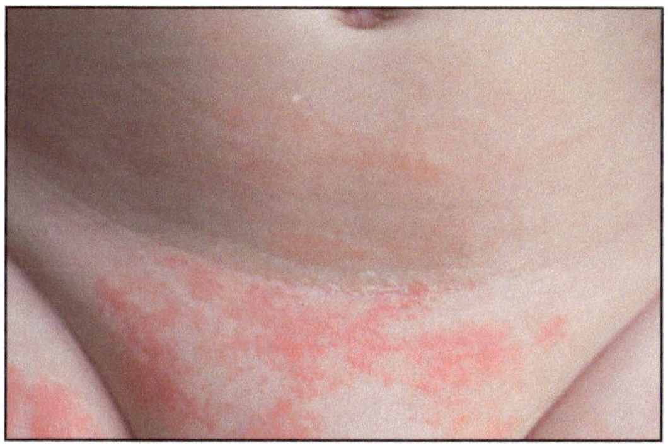

Contact Dermatitis:

Sx: Well demarcated erythema, erosions, vesicles, pruritis, burning

PE:

Dx:

____________________ Tx:

____

____

Folliculitis:

Sx: Erythematous papules or pustules involving hair follicles

PE:

Dx:

____________________ Tx:

____

____

Nummular Eczema: Coin shaped

Sx: Mostly on extremities

PE:

Dx:

Tx:

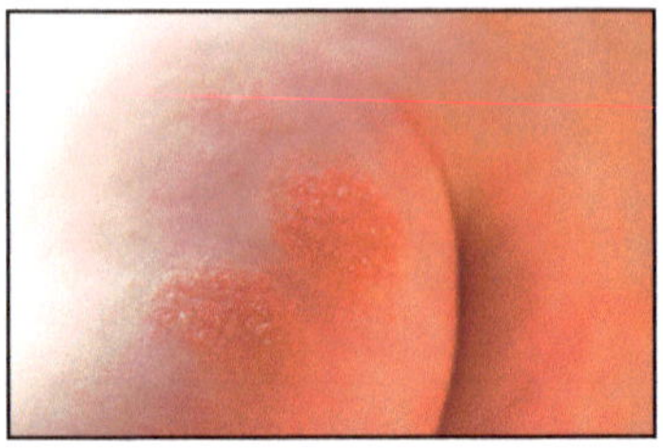

Perioral Dermatitis:

Sx: Papulopustular, plaques, scales around mouth (vermillion border is spared)

PE:

Dx:

Tx:

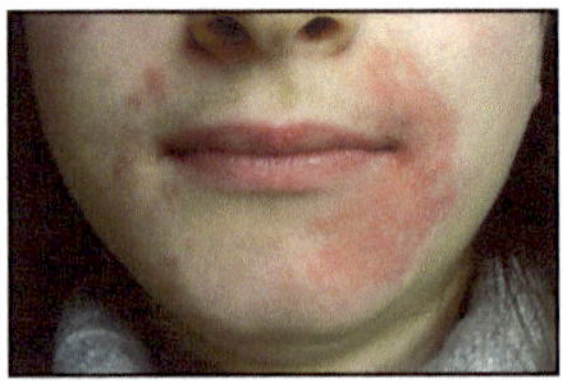

Dermatitis Herpetiform: **Associated w/celiac disease**

Sx: Autoimmune cutaneous eruption, gluten sensitivity

PE:

Dx: CBC and blood smear, tissue transglutaminase immunoglobulin A (tTg-IgA), skin biopsy, small bowel histology

Tx:

Pressure Ulcer:

Sx: Exudate, foul odor, localized tenderness

PE:

Dx:

Tx:

Seborrheic Dermatitis: **Cradle cap in infants**

Sx: Erythematous base. Yellow, greasy, scaly, patches, and crusted lesions

PE:

Dx:

Tx:

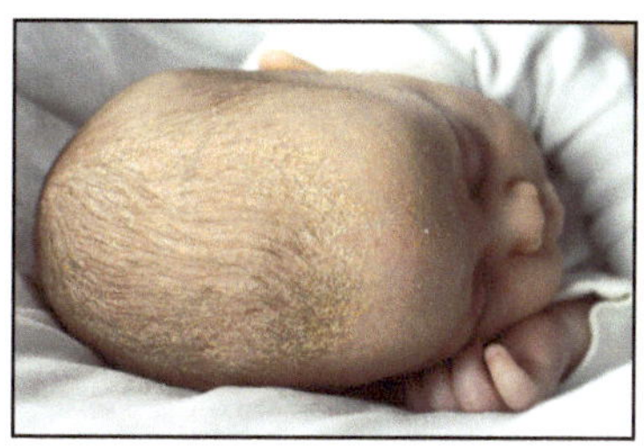

Drug Eruptions:

Common causes: NSAIDs

Sx: Erythematous, edematous plaque that leaves behind *hyperpigmented* macule

PE:

Dx:

Tx:

Vitiligo: Hypopigmentation

Co-occurring with pernicious anemia, autoimmune thyroiditis, Addison's, type 1 diabetes

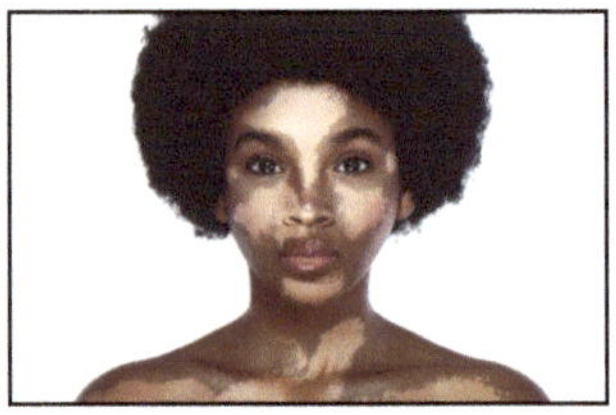

Sx:

PE:

Dx: Wood's light fluorescence over the lesion

Tx:

Melasma: Hyperpigmentation

Common causes: Estrongen, pregnancy, oral contraceptionn

Sx:

PE:

Dx:

Tx:

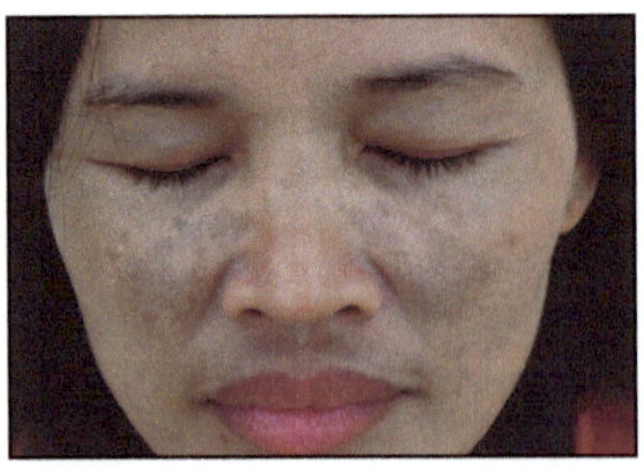

Rosacea: Rash, burns with certain foods (alcohol)

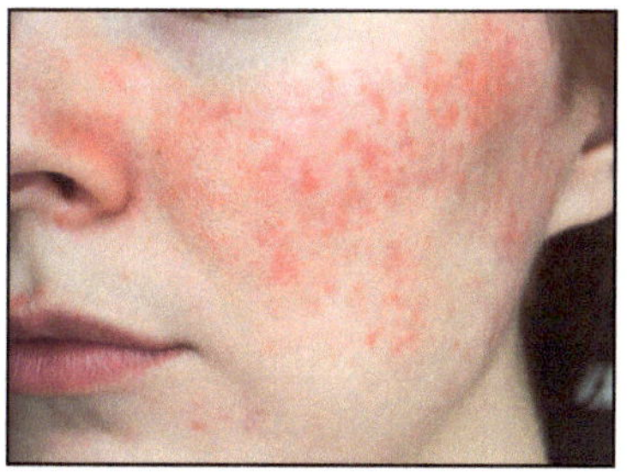

Sx: Flushing, erythema, telangiectasis, papules and pustules

PE:

Dx:

____

____

____

Tx:

Erysipelas: Lower extremities = Strep pyogenes
Face = Staph aureus

Sx: Abrupt onset, fever, chills, skin streaking with well defined margins (raised).

PE:

Dx:

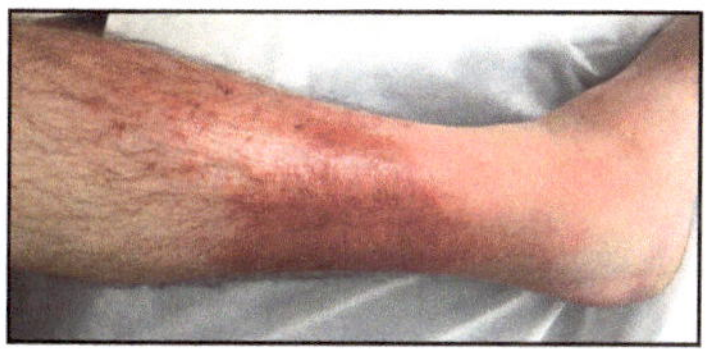

____

____

____

Tx:

Cellulitis: Staph & strep

Sx: Margins are NOT well demarcated, pain, erythema, warm, swelling

PE:

Dx:

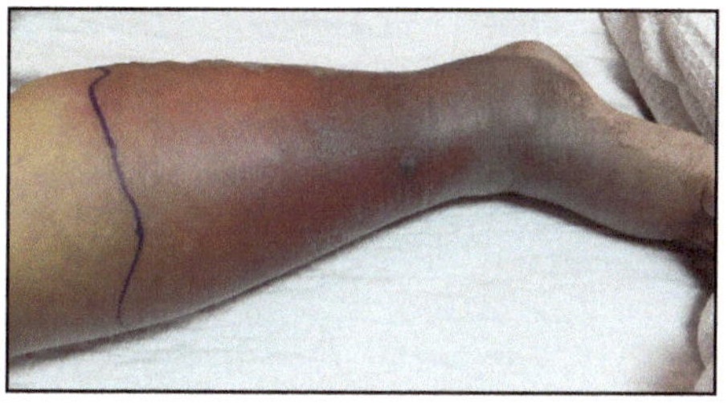

____

____

____

Tx:

Bullous Pemphigoid: **Chronic autoimmune, autoantibodies IgG**

Sx: Large fluid-filled bilsters

PE: Nikolsky

Dx:

Tx:

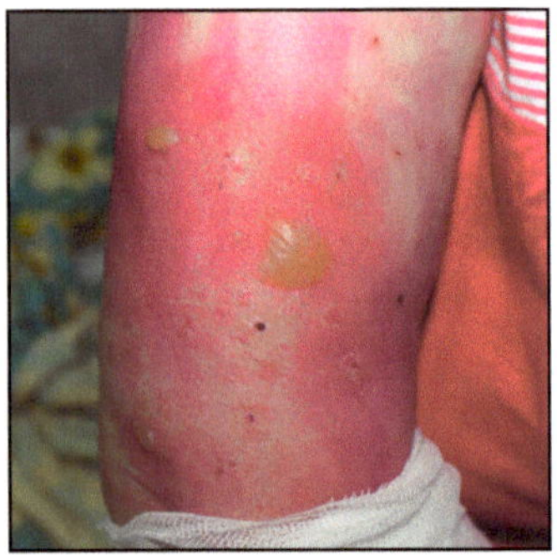

Pemphigus Vulgaris: **Autoimmune**

Sx: Blistering of skin and/or mucosa

PX:

Dx: Skin biopsy with direct immunofluorescence

Tx:

Simple Abscess: S. aureus – collection of pus within dermis and deeper tissue

Sx:

PE: Tender, erythematous, warm, fluctuant mass

Dx:

Tx:

Furuncle: S. aureus – infection of hair follicle

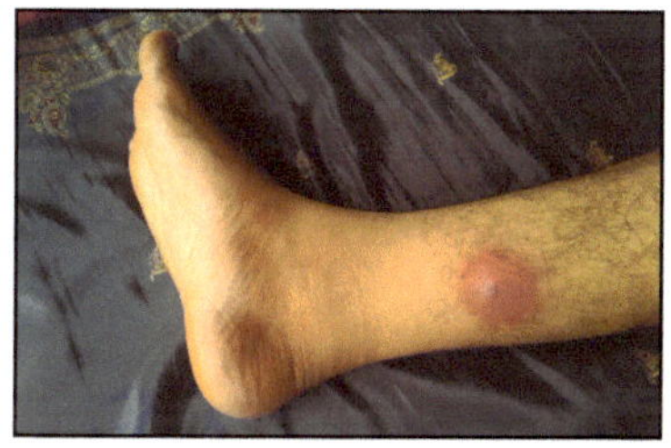

Sx:

PE: Nodule or pustule that may have purulent drainage or discharge

Dx:

Tx:

Carbuncle: S. aureus

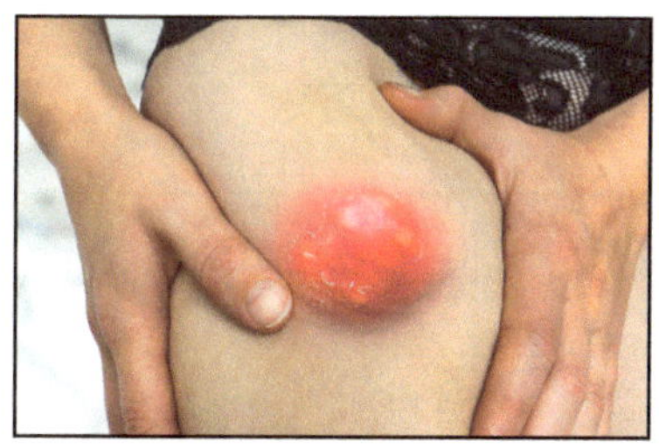

Sx:

PE: Cluster of furuncles connected at subcutaneous layer

Dx:

Tx:

Hidradenitis Suppurativa: **Chronic follicular occlusive disease. Smoking correlates with severity of disease**

Sx: Abscesses, sinus tracts, and scarring. Commonly in axillae, groin, and buttocks

PE:

Dx:

Tx:

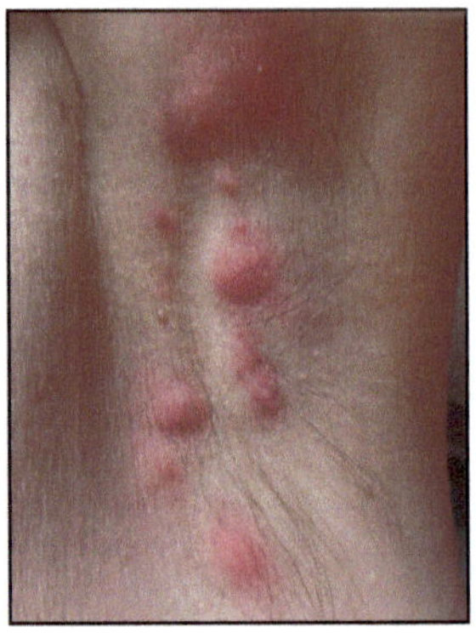

Pilonidal Disease:

Sx: Chronic follicle infection at the tailbone that contains hair and skin. Pain and swelling that comes and goes. Possible malodourous discharge

PE:

Dx:

Tx:

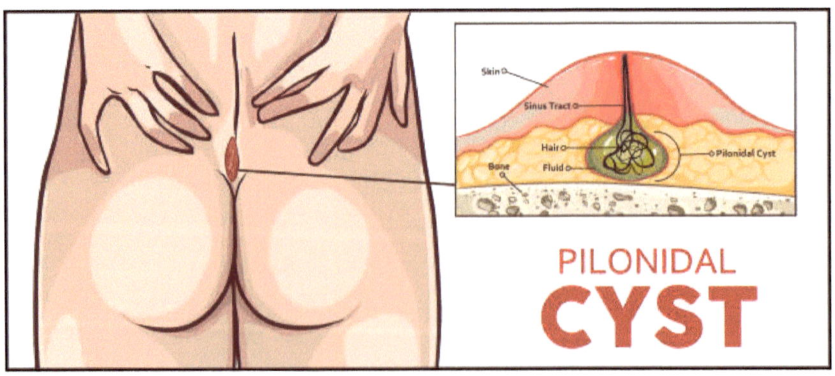

Stevens-Johnson Syndrome (SJS): Skin & mucous membranes: 3-10% of body

Toxic-Epidermal Necrolysis (TEN): More than 30% of body

Sx: Rash, mucosal involvement

- Prodrome: Flu-like symptoms
- Painful, red or purplish rash that spreads, blisters
- Associated with anticonvulsant meds, infection, antibiotic use, lupus, AIDS

PE:

Dx: Skin biopsy:

____

____

____

Tx:

Scalded Skin Syndrome: **Exfoliative toxin by S. aureus (spares mucous membranes)**

Sx: Prodrome, fever, rapid progression of erythema in shin folds, pain

PE:

Dx: Bacterial culture

Tx:

Drug Reaction with Eosinophilia and Systemic Symptoms (DRESS)

Common causes: Anticonvulsant (carbamazepine), allopurinol, sulfonamides, antibiotic

Sx: Skin eruption, fever, facial edema, visceral involvement, blood involvement

PE:

Dx:

Tx:

Fungi or Dermatophytes

Epidermomycosis = Skin - Trichomycosis = Hair & hair follicles - Onychomycosis = Nails

Tinea Pedis: "Athlete's foot"

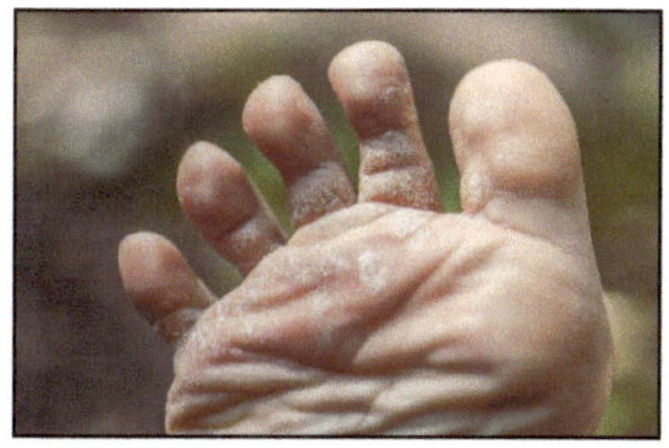

Sx:

PE:

Dx: Potassium hydroxide (KOH)

____

____

____

Tx:

Tinea Cruris: "Jock itch"

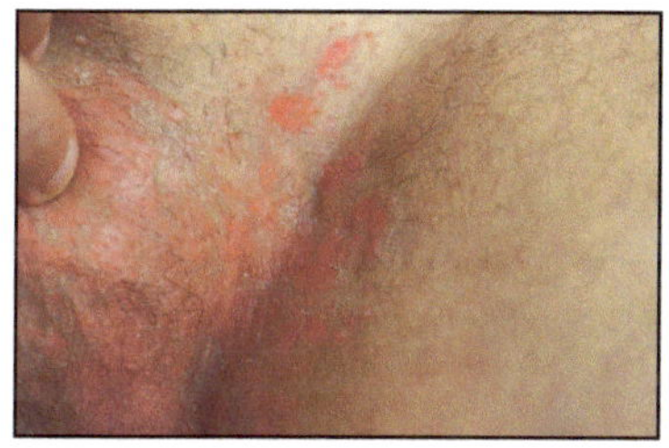

Sx:

PE:

Dx: Potassium hydroxide (KOH)

____

____

____

Tx:

Tinea Capitis (Pediculosis Capitis):

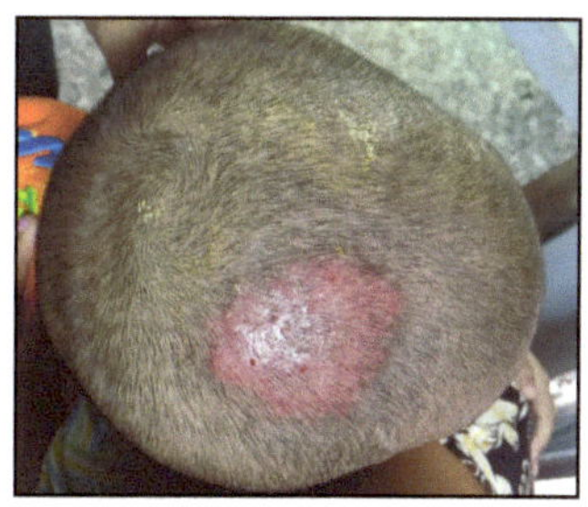

Sx: Patchy alopecia, scaling lesion with central clearing

PE:

Dx:

____

____

____

Tx:

Tinea Corporis:

Sx: Well demarcated scaling plaques with central clearing

PE:

Dx: Potassium hydroxide (KOH) prep

Tx:

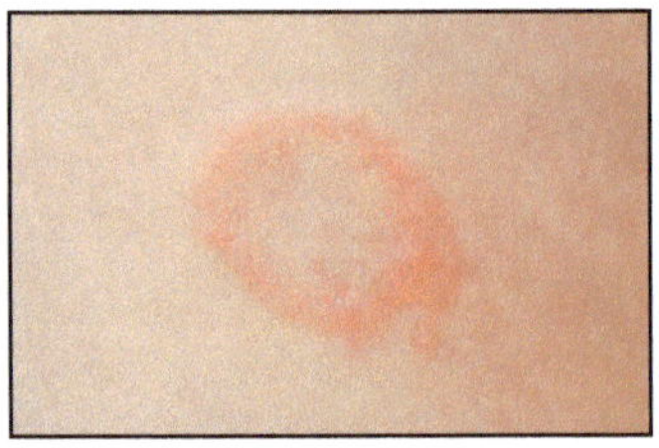

Tinea Versicolor: Hypopigmentation caused by fungus (Malassezia furfur)

Sx: Scaly patches on chest & trunk, may have mild itching

PE:

Dx:

Tx:

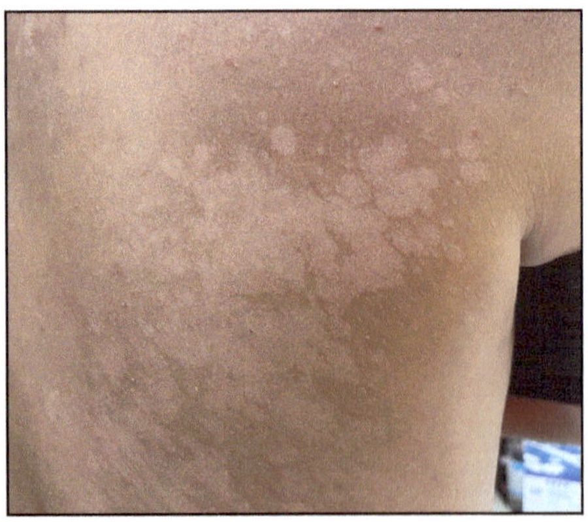

Tinea Barbae: Fungal infection caused by dermatophytes

Sx:

PE:

Dx:

Tx:

Onychomycosis:

Sx: Nail fungus causing thickened, brittle, crumbly nails

PE:

Dx: KOH prep or Periodic Acid-Schiff

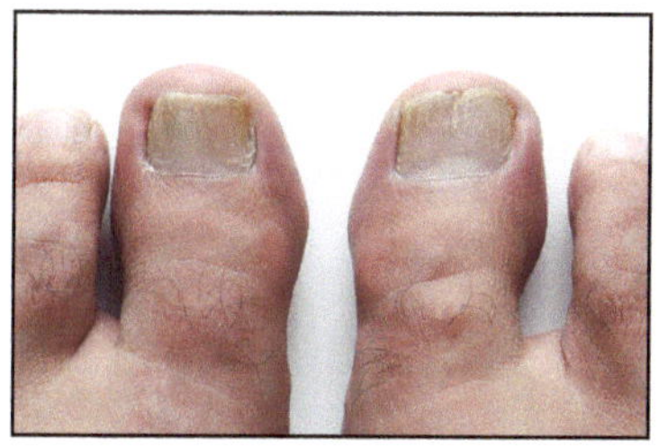

Tx:

Verrucae

Verruca Vulgaris (Common Wart):

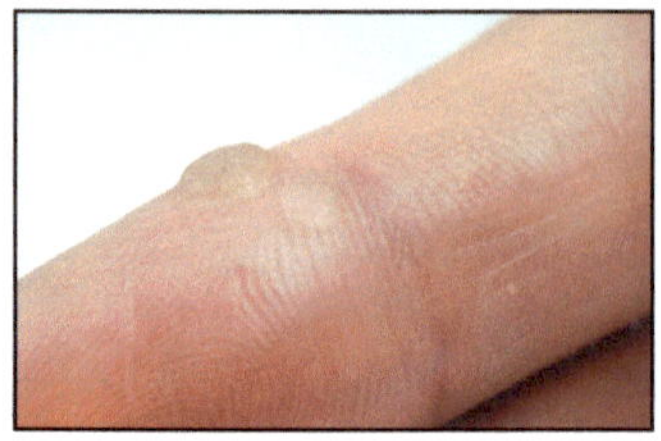

Sx: Round, raised papule with tiny black dots

PE:

Dx:

Tx:

Verruca Plana (Flat Wart):

Sx: Flat topped, slightly raised

PX:

Dx:

Tx:

Verrucae Plantaris (Plantar Wart):

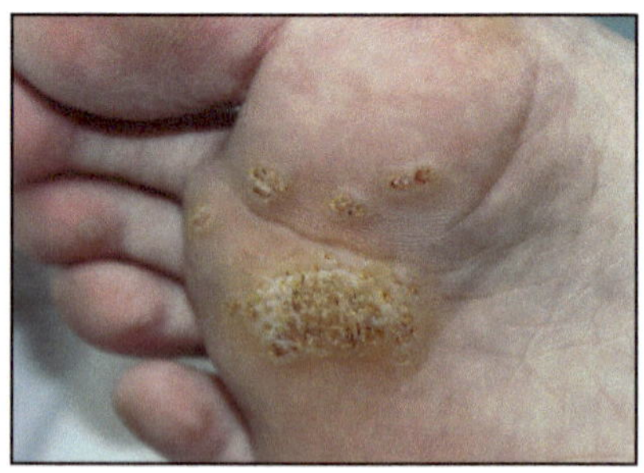

Sx:

PE: Hyperkeratotic debris with thrombosed capillaries

Dx:

Tx: Salicylic acid, cryotherapy

Condyloma Acuminatum (Venereal Warts):

Risk Factors: Early age for intercourse, increased amount of sexual partners

Sx: Lesions 1-3 cm, sessile, papillomas that may coalesce into larger cauliflower like lesions

PE:

Dx:

____

____

____

Tx:

Hair Loss (Alopecias)

Alopecia Areata: **"Exclamation point hairs"**

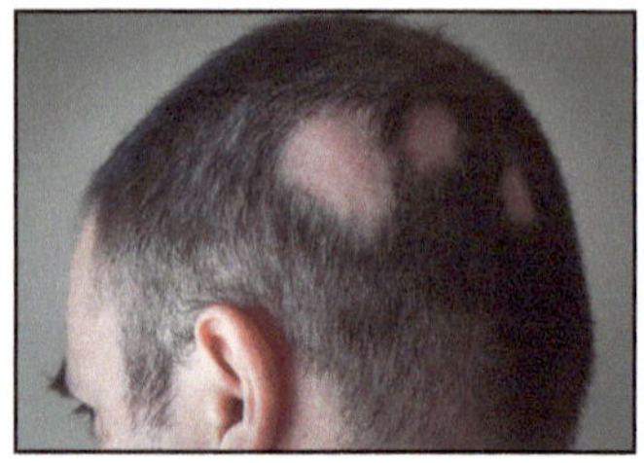

Risk Factors: Hashimoto's, Addison's, vitiligo, pernicious anemia

Sx: Smooth, non-scaring

PE:

Dx: Pull test, clinical

____________________ **Tx:**

____

____

Traction Alopecia:

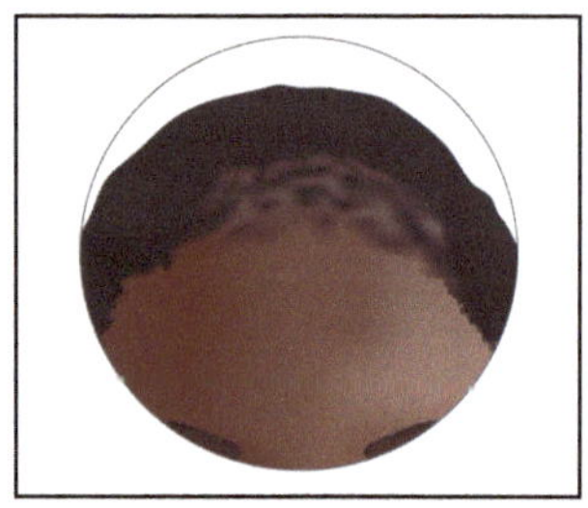

Sx:

PE:

Dx: Clinical

____________________ **Tx:**

____

____

Telogen Effluvium: Psychological or physiological stress

Sx: Temporary thinning of hair

PE:

Dx:

Tx:

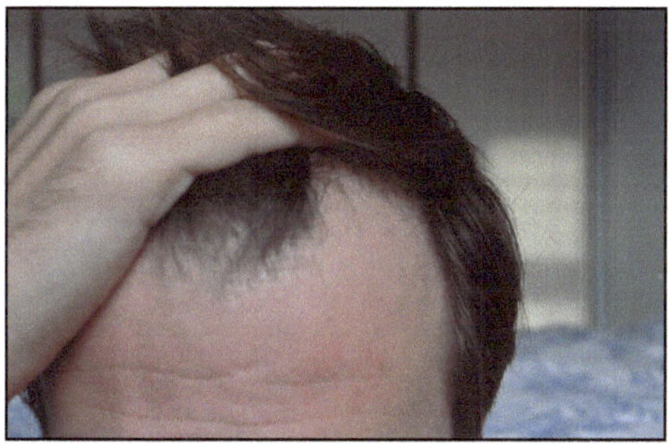

Androgenic Alopecia: Male pattern baldness

Sx: Gradual receding hairline

PE:

Dx: Negative hair pull test, thyroid function, serum ferritin

Tx:

Pediatric Derm Concerns

Erythema Infectiosum (Fifth Disease): **Parvo B19**

Sx: "Slapped cheek" spares nose and mouth. Lacy reticular rash on extremities that SPARES PALMS & SOLES

PE:

Dx:

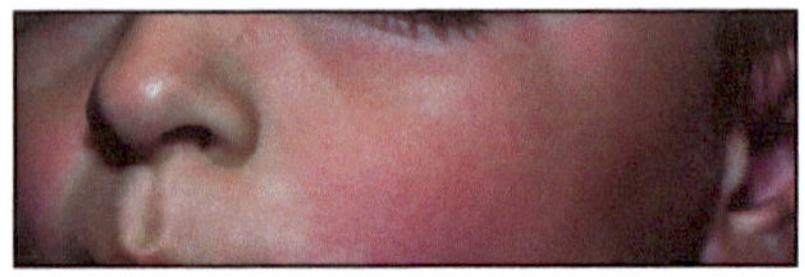

Tx:

Hand, Foot, and Mouth (Coxsackie Virus): **Respiratory droplets, summer & fall months**

Sx:

PE:

Dx: Viral culture, CBC

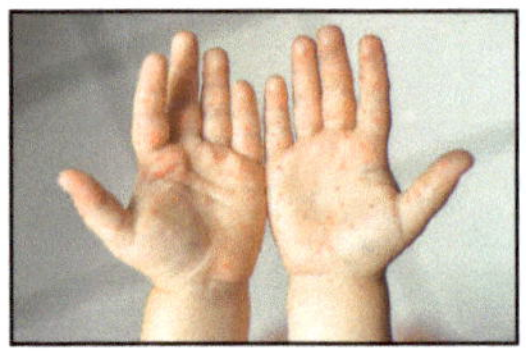

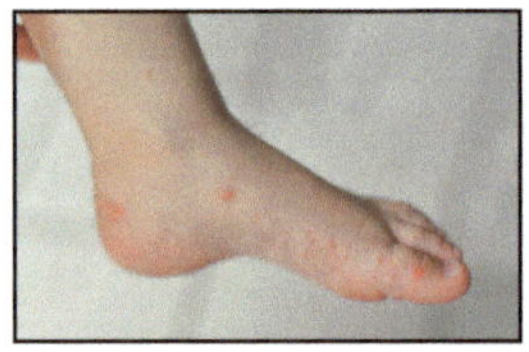

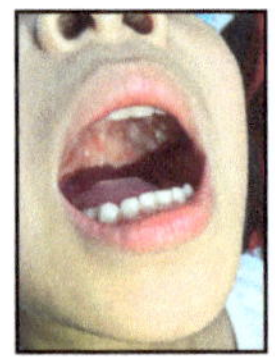

Tx:

Measles (Rubeola):

Sx: 4 C's: Cough, coryza, conjunctivitis, cephalocaudal morbilliform rash
Rash starts at hairline then moves to palms & soles of feet
Rash lasts 7 days.
Kolpik spots - small, erythematous spots on buccal mucosa with blue/white pale center, usually precedes rash by 1-2 days

PE:

Dx:

Tx:

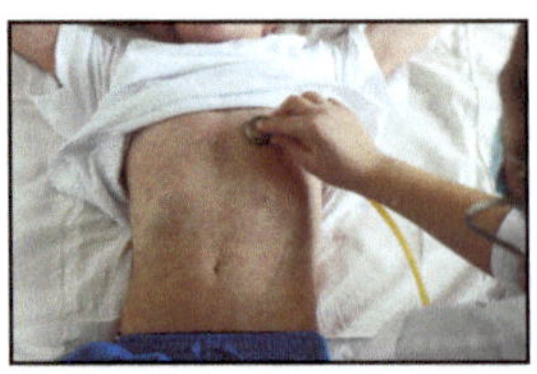

Rubella (German Measles):

Sx: Fever, maculopapular rash, postauricular lymphadenopathy

3-day rash: pink, spotted maculopapular rash ***first on face then to trunk & extremities***

Pregnant women should avoid exposure

PE:

Dx:

______________________________ **Tx:**

____

____

Congenital Rubella: Microcephaly, ophthalmologist issues

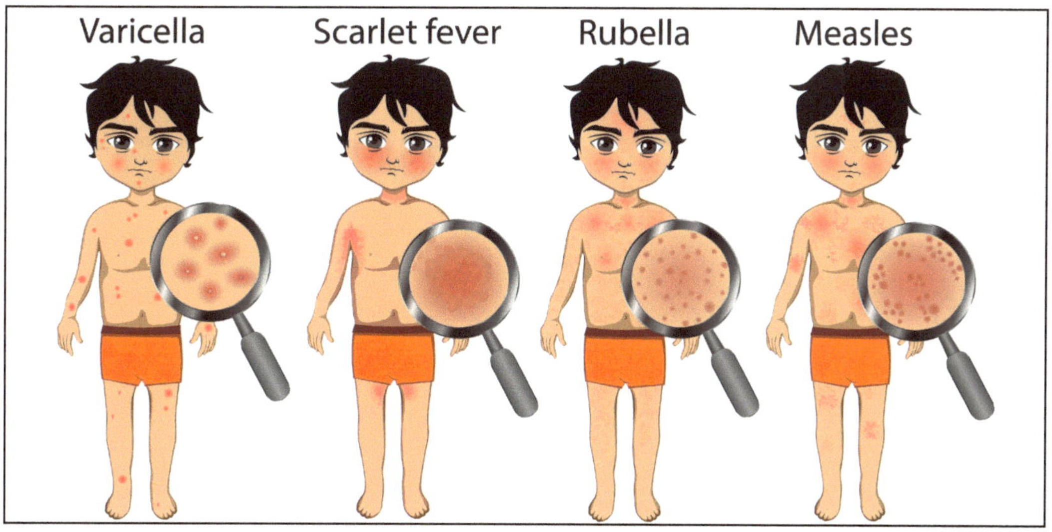

Impetigo: S. aureus

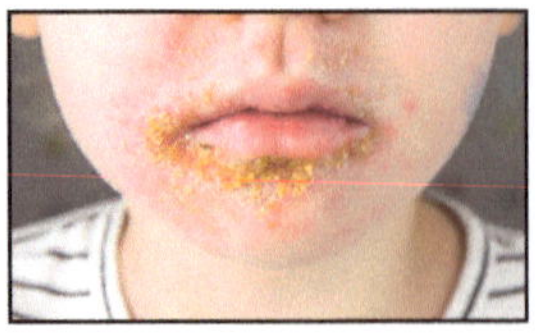

Sx: Honey crusted lesions

PE:

Dx:

Tx:

Molluscum Contagiosum: Poxvirus

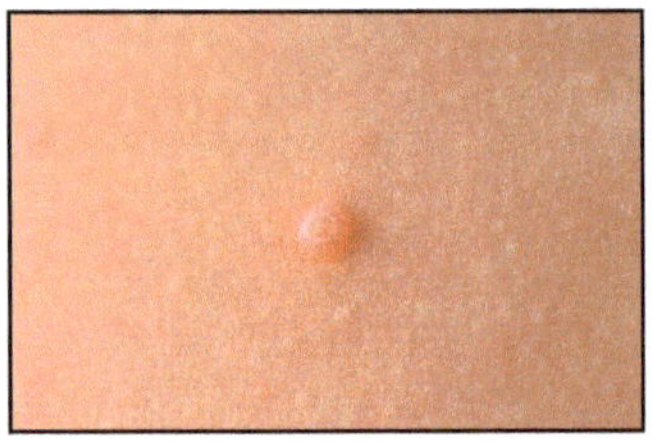

Sx: Pearly papules with umbilication

PE:

Dx:

Tx:

Lice:

Sx: Scalp itching, visible eggs

PE:

Dx: Clinical

Tx:

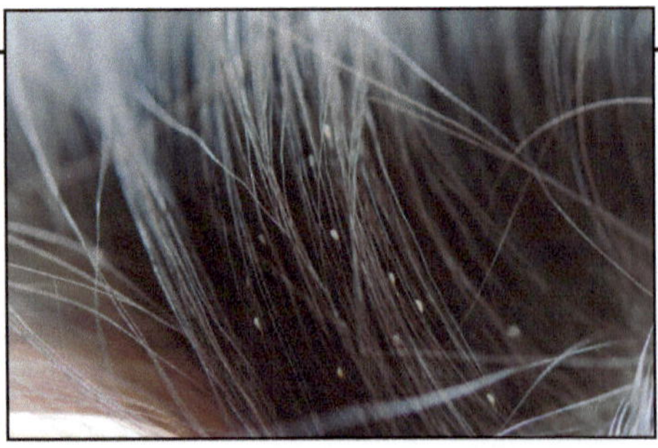

Scabies:

Sx: Pruritic papules in an "s" shaped or linear pattern (burrows). Usually affects web spaces of hands, wrists, and waist. Itching that is worse at night

PE:

Dx:

Tx:

Scabies

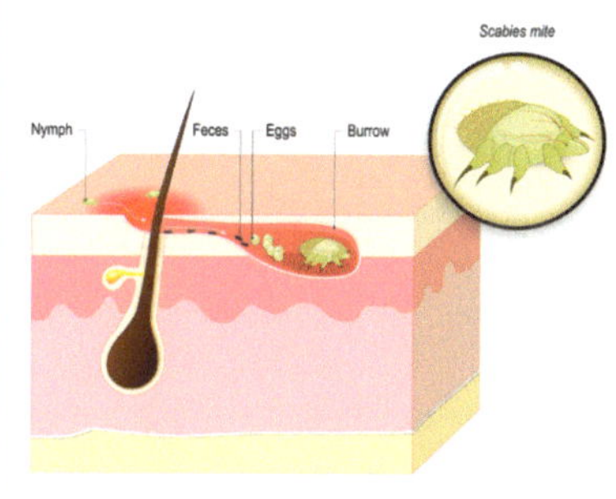

Erythemas

Erythema Multiforme: HSV (most common) and sulfa drugs

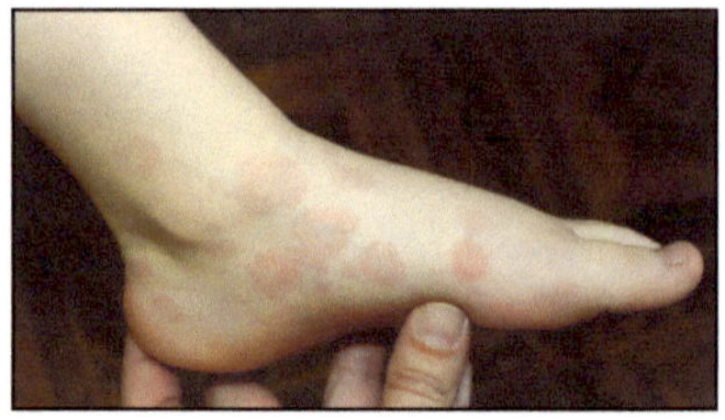

Sx: Target shaped, blanching, does not itch

PE:

Dx: CBC, HSV serology, PCR

Tx:

Erythema Marginatum: Associated with rheumatic fever

Sx: Macule with central clearing that the spares face

PE:

Dx:

Tx:

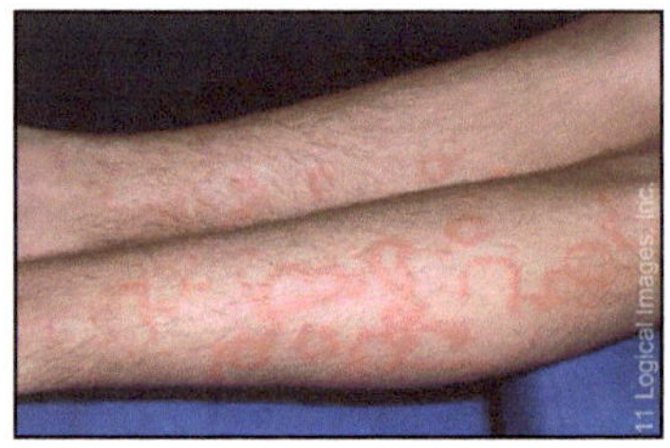

Erythema Nodosum:

Cause: Infection, autoimmune, medications, pregnancy, inflammatory conditions (Sarcoidosis, Crohn's)

Sx: Inflammatory nodules

PE:

Dx:

Tx:

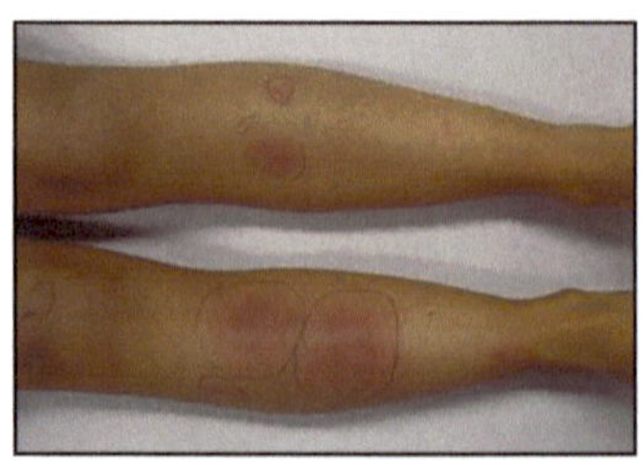

Spider Bites

Brown Recluse:

Sx: Necrotic wound

PE:

Dx:

Tx:

Black Widow:

Sx: Neurologic manifestations

PE:

Dx:

Tx:

Dermatologic Carcinomas

Actinic Keratosis: **Most common cause sun exposure - PRE-CANCER**

Sx: Single or multiple scaly macules or papules

PE:

Dx:

Tx:

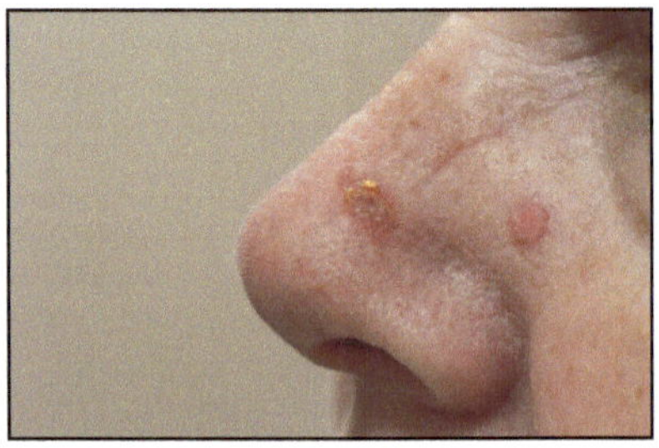

Squamous Cell Carcinoma: **Actinic keratosis is precursor**

Sx: Nonhealing lesion, may bleed. Location: Sun-exposed areas

PE:

Dx:

Tx:

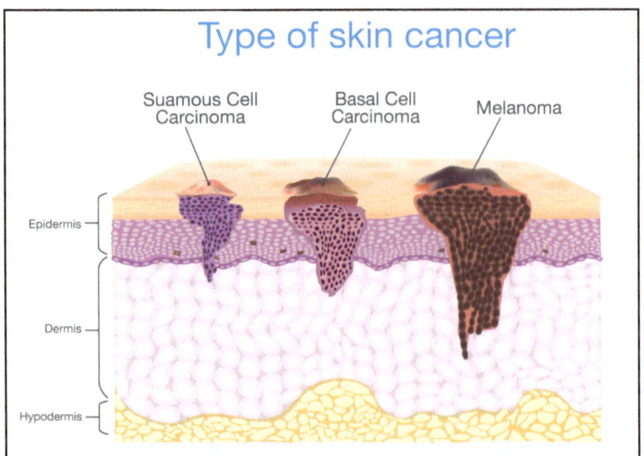

Melanoma:

Sx: Asymmetry, border irregularity, color variations, diameter > 6mm

PE:

Dx:

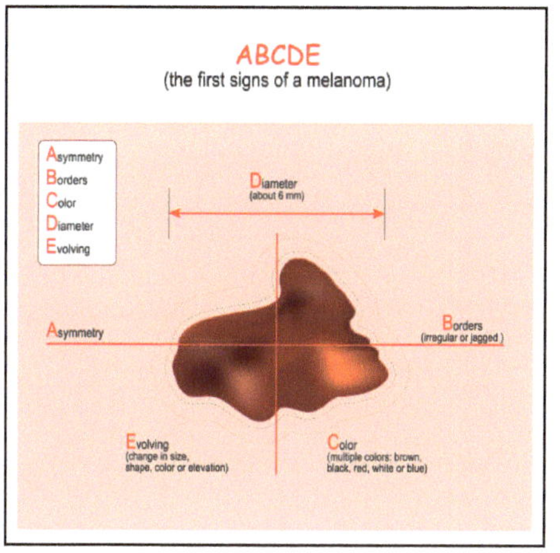

Tx:

Basal Cell Carcinoma: Most common skin cancer

Sx: Pearly nodule, "rolled" raised edge, telangiectasis, non-healing scabs, ulcerated center with pearly heaped edges

PE:

Dx:

Tx:

Acne

Acne:

Sx: Uninflamed blackheads, pustules, large erythematous and tender bumps

PE:

Dx:

Tx:

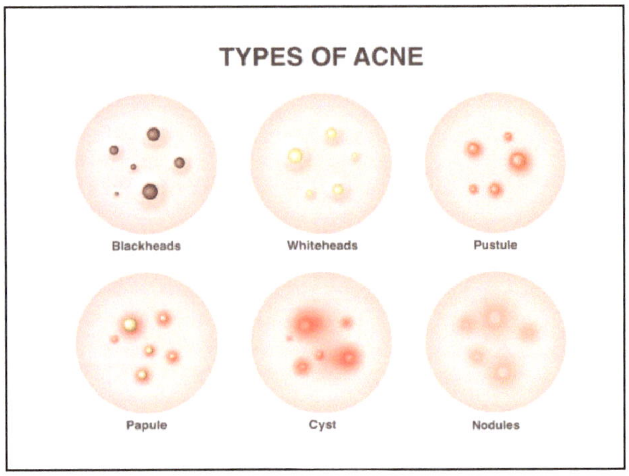

Acne Vulgaris:

Sx:

PE: Comedones, inflamed nodules

Dx: Clinical

Tx:

Misc. Derm

Seborrheic Keratosis:

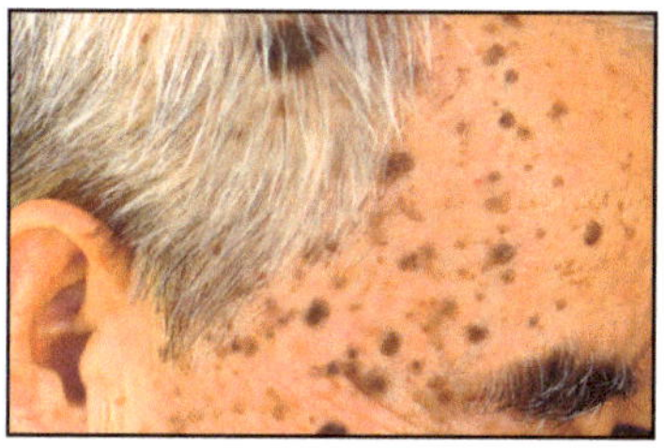

Sx: Yellow or light to dark brown lesions, raised, waxy, painless

PE:

Dx:

Tx:

Erythrasma:

Sx: Sharply delineated, dry, brown, scaling patches (axillae, genitocrural creases)

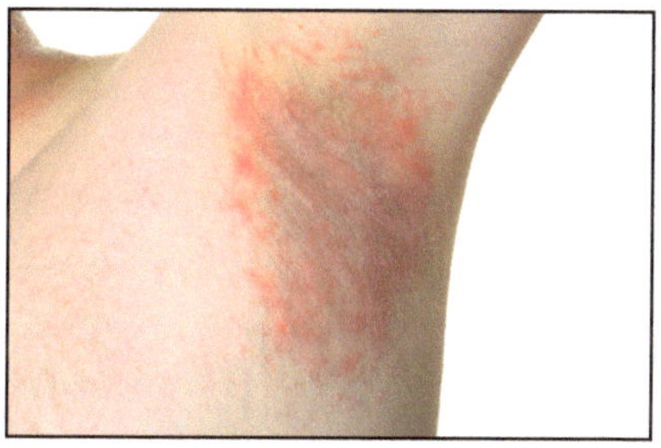

PE:

Dx:

Tx:

Pityriasis Rosea: **Self-limiting**

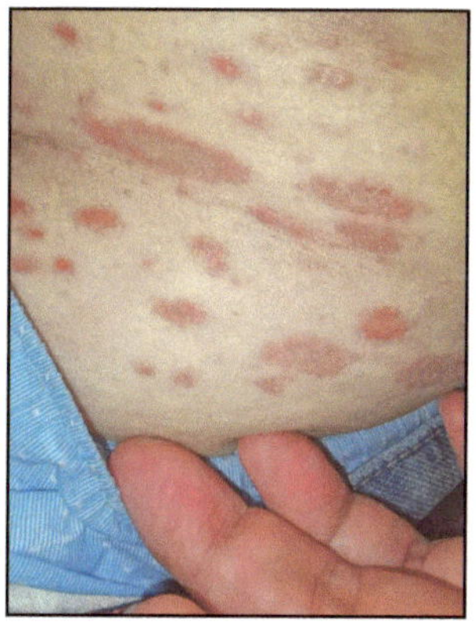

Sx: Herald Patch, central clearing with Christmas tree distribution (Langer's lines), salmon-colored patches

PE:

Dx:

Tx:

Dog Bite:

Sx: Laceration

PE:

Dx: Clinical

Tx:

Cat Bite: **Pasteurella most common bacteria**

Sx: Laceration, puncture wounds

PE:

Dx: Clinical

Tx:

Cherry Angioma:

Sx: Flat, small, red

PE:

Dx:

Tx:

Solar Lentigo: **Liver spots**

Sx:

PE:

Dx: Skin biopsy

Tx:

Sebaceous Cyst: **Blocked gland or duct**

Sx: Can range in size

PE:

Dx:

Tx:

Keloids: Abnormal scarring

Sx:

PE:

Dx: Clinical

Tx:

Lipoma:

Sx: Slow growing and usually harmless

PE:

Dx: X-ray, MRI, or biopsy to rule out other causes

Tx:

Burns

Rule of 9's

***Paronychia:* In MSK**

***Roseola (6th disease) (Herpesvirus 6 or 7):* In ID**

***Felon:* In MSK**

***Genital Herpes:* In ID**

***Erythema Migrans (Lyme Disease):* In ID**

Medications

________________: MOA = ________________________________

Indication(s)=____________________________________

Side Effects = ____________________________________

Types/ Examples = ________________________________

____

____

________________: MOA = ________________________________

Indication(s)=____________________________________

Side Effects = ____________________________________

Types/ Examples = ________________________________

____

____

________________: MOA = ________________________________

Indication(s)=____________________________________

Side Effects = ____________________________________

Types/ Examples = ________________________________

____

____

________________: MOA = ________________________________

Indication(s)=____________________________________

Side Effects = ____________________________________

Types/ Examples = ________________________________

____

____

________________: MOA = ________________________________

Indication(s)=____________________________________

Side Effects = ____________________________________

Types/ Examples = ________________________________

____

____

Medications

______________: MOA = ______________

Indication(s)=______________

Side Effects = ______________

Types/ Examples = ______________

____

____

______________: MOA = ______________

Indication(s)=______________

Side Effects = ______________

Types/ Examples = ______________

____

____

______________: MOA = ______________

Indication(s)=______________

Side Effects = ______________

Types/ Examples = ______________

____

____

______________: MOA = ______________

Indication(s)=______________

Side Effects = ______________

Types/ Examples = ______________

____

____

______________: MOA = ______________

Indication(s)=______________

Side Effects = ______________

Types/ Examples = ______________

____

____

Endocrinology

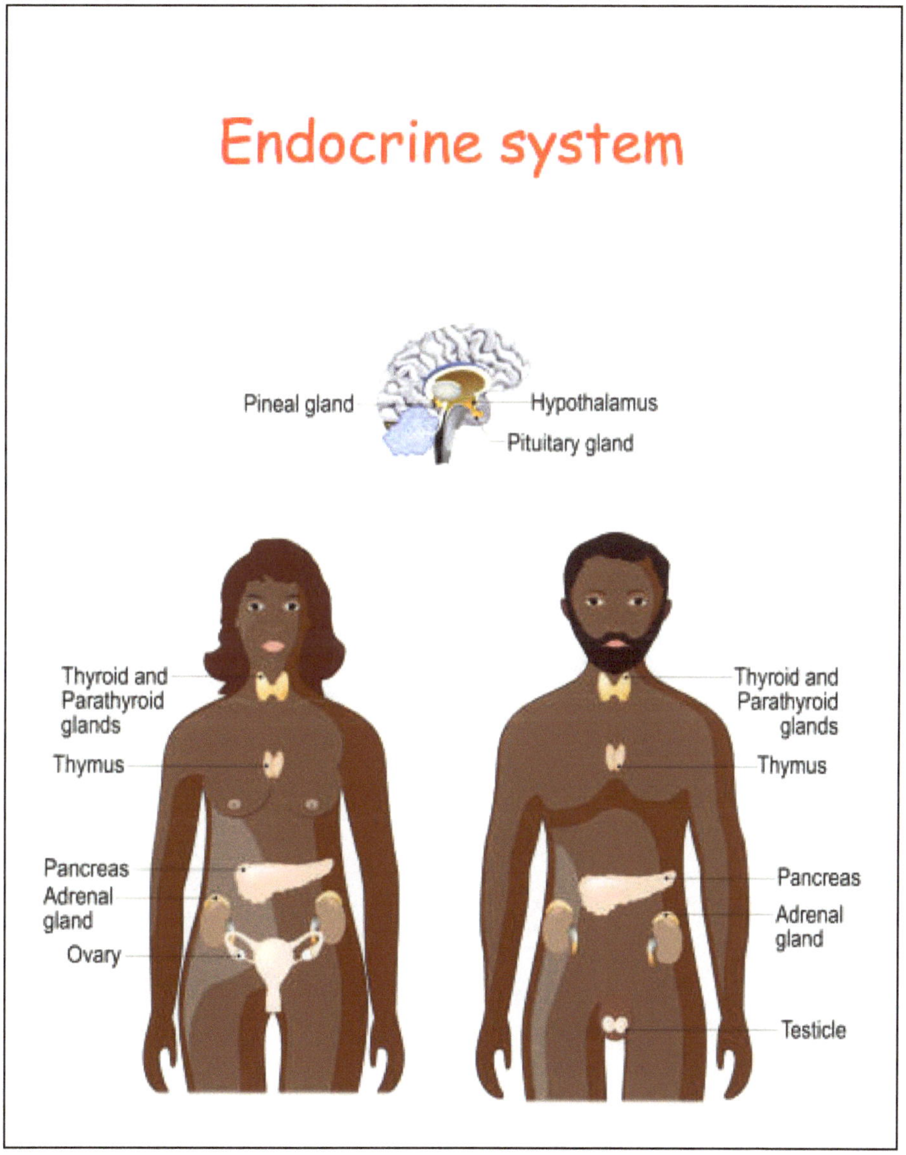

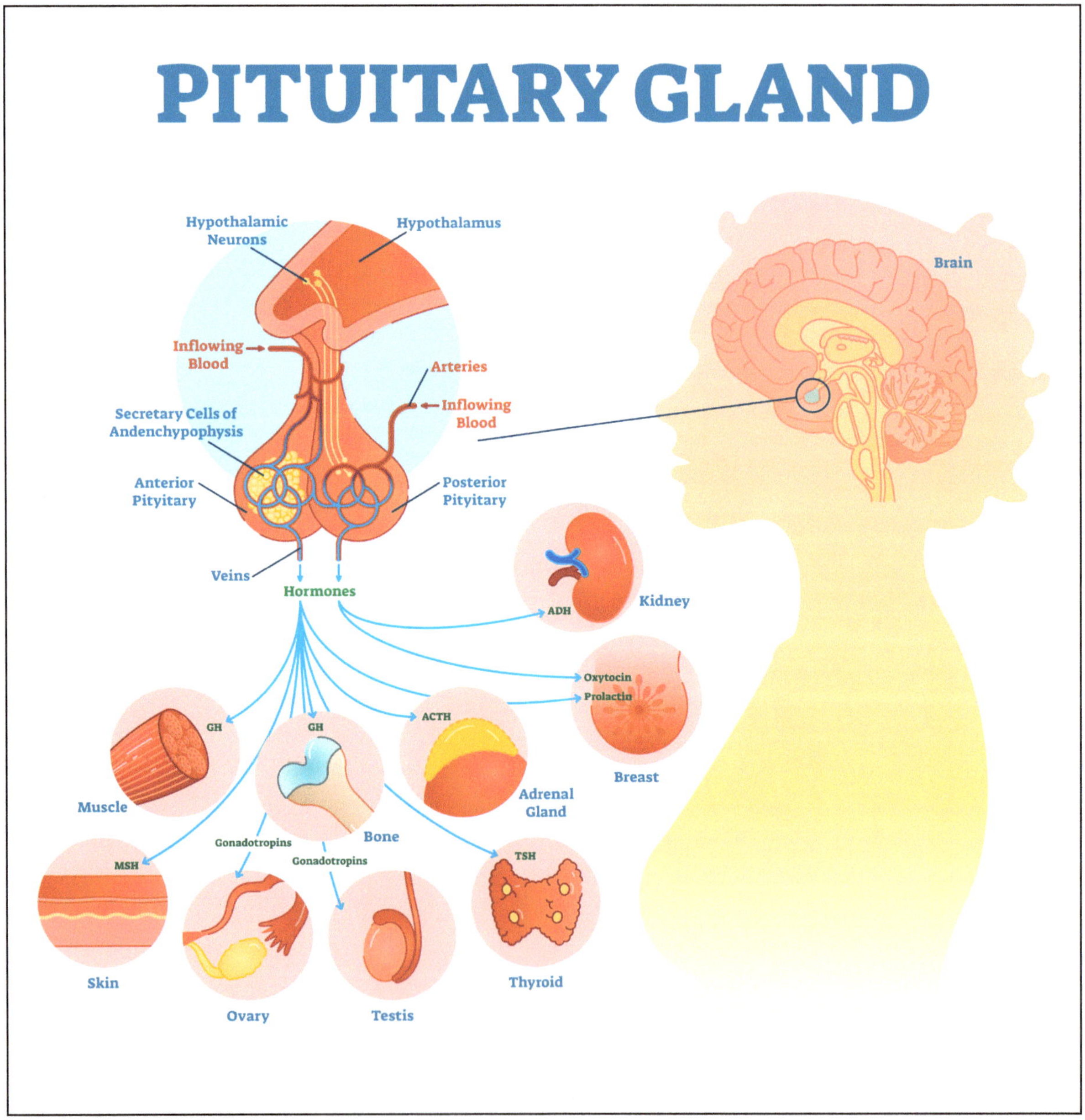
PITUITARY GLAND
Hypothalamic Neurons
Hypothalamus
Brain
Inflowing Blood
Arteries
Inflowing Blood
Secretary Cells of Andenchypophysis
Anterior Pityitary
Posterior Pityitary
Veins
Hormones
ADH
Kidney
Oxytocin
Prolactin
Breast
GH
GH
ACTH
Muscle
Adrenal Gland
Bone
Gonadotropins
Gonadotropins
MSH
TSH
Skin
Ovary
Testis
Thyroid

Thyroid Disorders

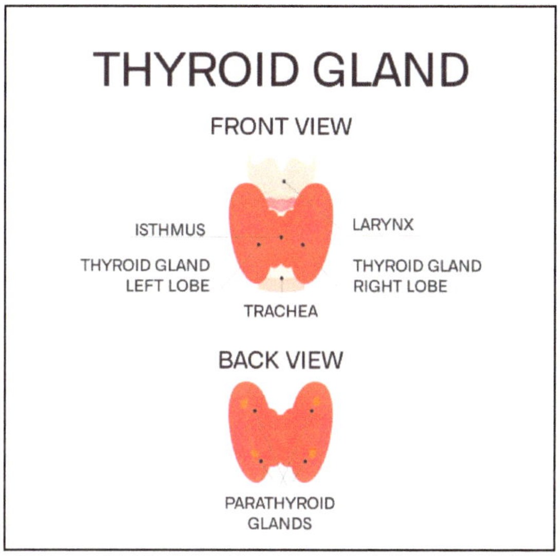

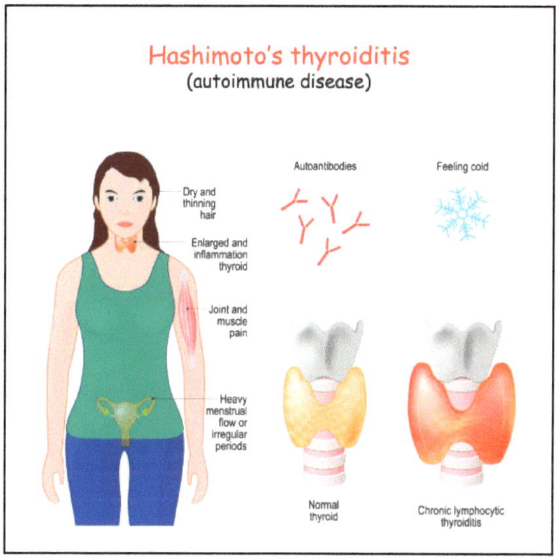

Hypothyroidism:
Hashimoto's:

Sx: Cold intolerance, dry skin, fatigue, constipation, hair loss

PE:

Dx: Increase TSH, decrease T3 & T4, + anti-thyroid peroxidase AB, + anti-thyroglobin Ab

______________________________ **Tx:**

____

____

Myxedema: **Extreme form of hypothyroidism**

Sx: Bradycardia, hypothermia, hypoglycemia

PE:

Dx:

______________________________ **Tx:**

____

____

Hyperthyroidism:

Sx: Heat intolerance, weight loss, hyperactivity, diarrhea, tachycardia

PE:

Dx: Decreased TSH

Tx:

Graves' Disease: Most common cause of hyperthyroidism

Sx:

PE:

Dx: Decreased TSH, increased T3 & T4

Tx:

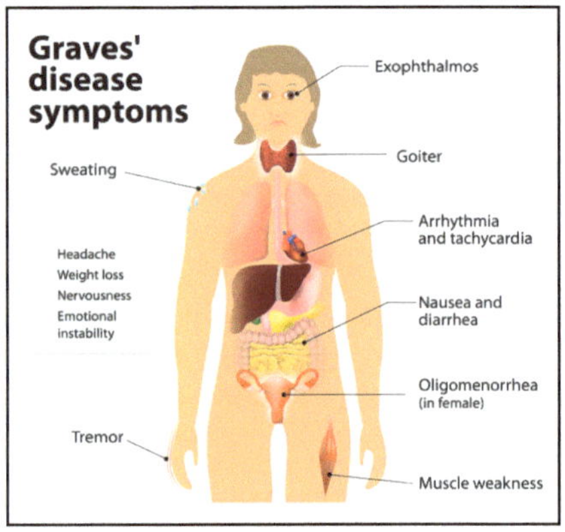

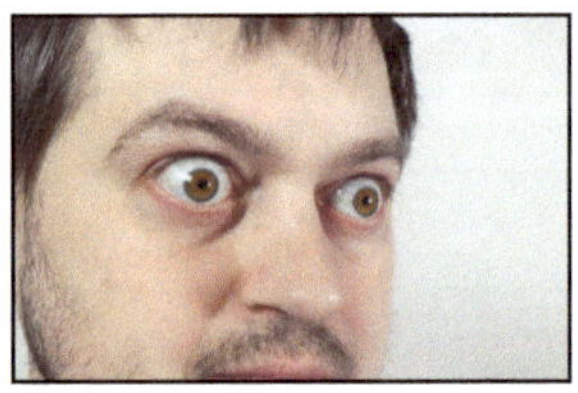

Thyroid Storm: Extreme form of hyperthyroidism

Sx: Palpitations, high fever, nausea, vomiting, psychosis, tremors

PE:

Dx:

Tx:

Thyroid Nodule:

Sx: Most often asymptomatic

PE:

Dx: Fine needle aspiration with biopsy

Tx:

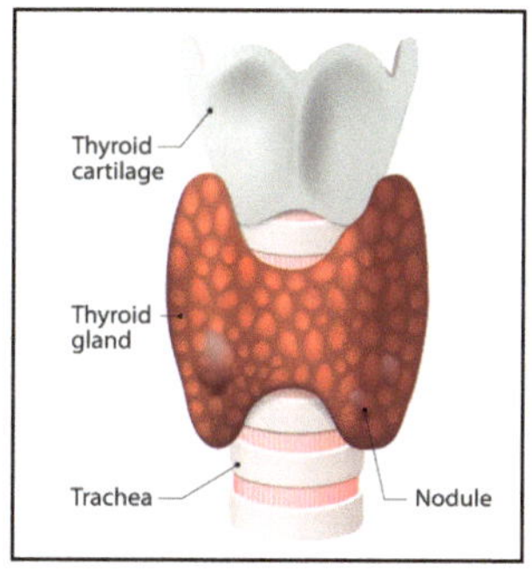

Thyroid Cancer:

Papillary (most common, good prognosis)

Follicular (good prognosis)

Medullary (MEN2, poor prognosis)

Anaplastic (worst prognosis)

Sx:

PE:

Dx:

Tx:

Thyroid Medications:

Hyperthyroid:

Methimazole:

PTU:

Propranolol:

Iodides:

Radioactive Iodine:

Hypothyroid:

Levothyroxine:

Parathyroid Disorders

Low serum Ca - Parathyroid glands - PTH - bones & kidneys

PTH at bones stimulates osteoclasts to break down bone

PTH at kidneys stimulates calcitriol (vit D) release – small intestines absorb more Ca

---

Hyperparathyroidism:

Sx: Stones, bones, moans, groans (kidney stones, bone pain, myalgia, fatigue)

PE:

Dx:

Tx:

Hypoparathyroidism:

Most common cause: Thyroidectomy

Sx: Tetany, spasms, cramps

PE:

Dx:

Tx:

Adrenal Gland Disorders

Hypothalamus - CRH – Anterior pit - ACTH – Adrenal cortex – Cortisol - Adrenal medulla - Catecholamines (EPI & NorEPI)

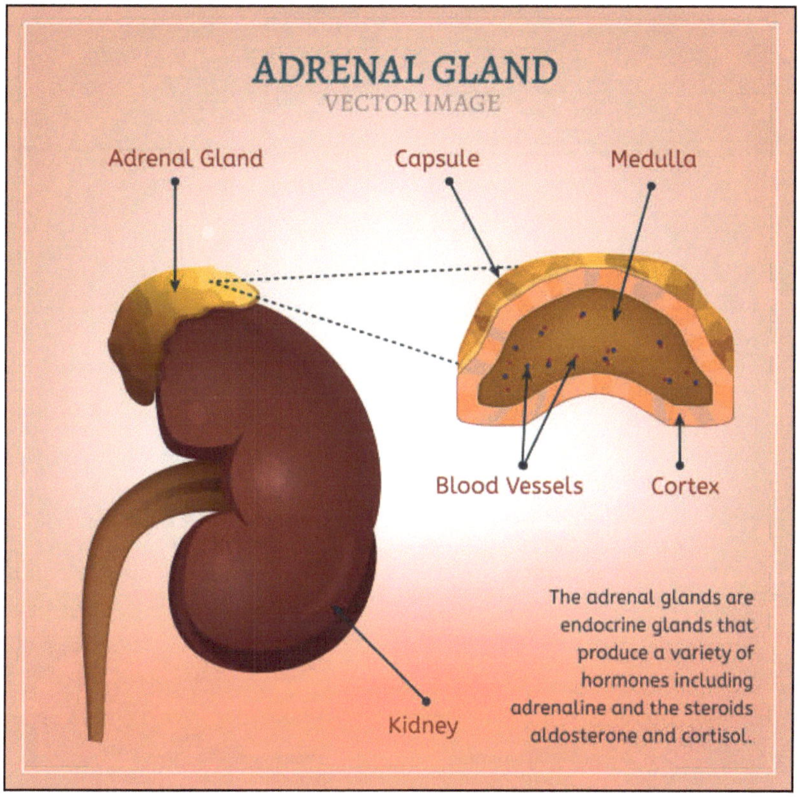

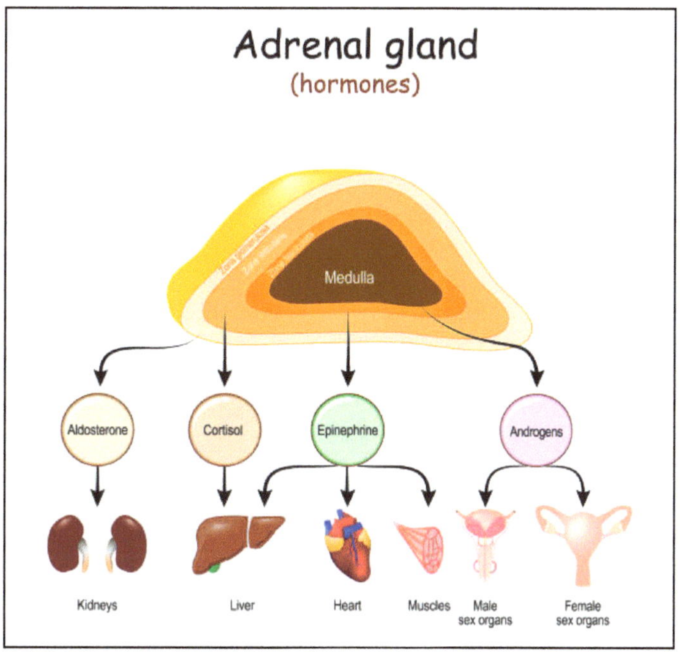

Cushing's Disease/Syndrome:

Causes:

Sx:

PE: Moon face, buffalo hump

Dx:

___

___

___

Tx:

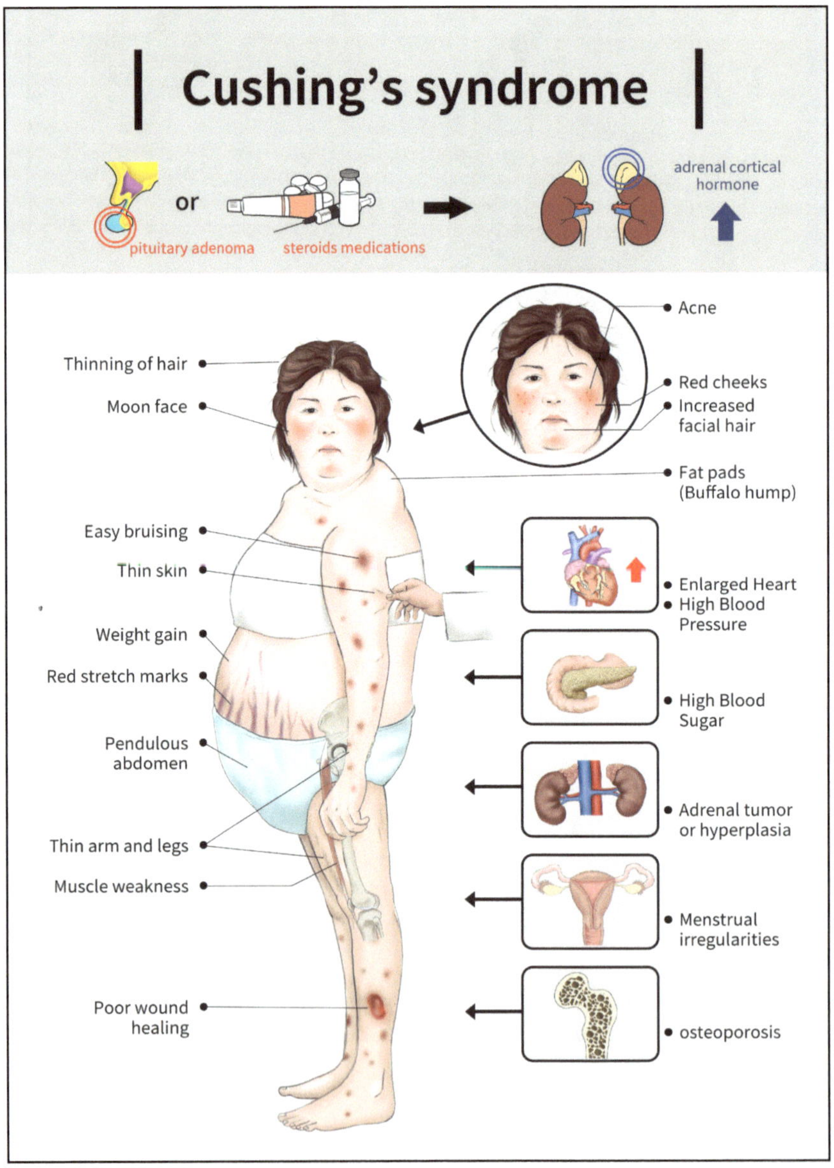

Addison's Disease:

Causes:

Sx:

PE: Hyperpigmentation (JFK)

Dx:

Tx:

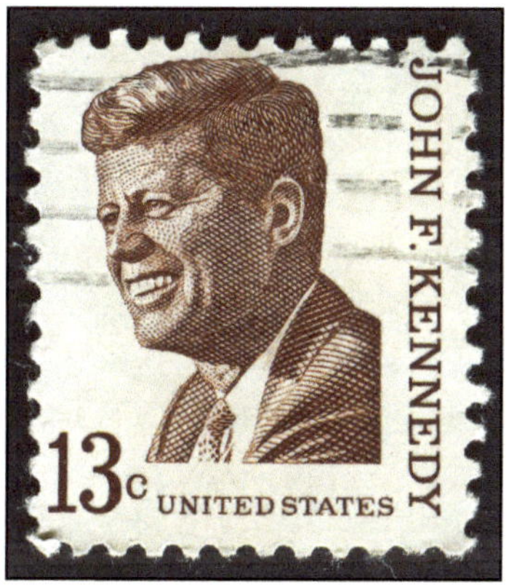

Pheochromocytoma: **Adrenal catecholamine secreting tumor**

Sx:

PE: Resistant hypertension, palpitations, headaches, excessive sweating

Dx:

Tx:

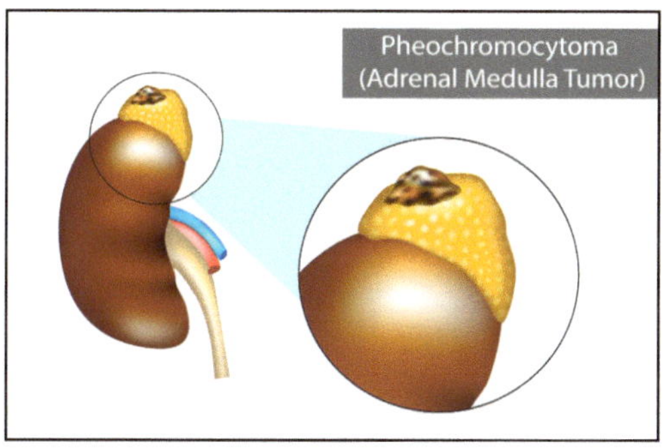

Pituitary Gland Disorders

Syndrome of Inappropriate Antidiuretic Hormone (SIADH):

Causes: Pituitary trauma, tumor (lung or GI)

Sx: Symptoms of hyponatremia, concentrated urine

PE:

Dx:

______________________________ Tx:

____

____

Diabetes Insipidus (DI):

Central DI: Pituitary/hypothalamus (decreased ADH production)

Sx:

PE:

Dx: Fluid deprivation test = continued dilute urine. Desmopressin stimulation = decreased urine output and increased urine osmolality

Nephrogenic DI: Kidney (insensitivity to ADH)

Sx:

PE:

Dx: Fluid deprivation test = continued dilute urine. Desmopressin stimulation = continued dilute urine

______________________________ Tx:

____

____

Acromegaly (Adults)/Giantism (Children):

Most common cause: Pituitary adenoma

Sx:

PE:

Dx: Increase in insulin-like growth factor 1 (IGF-1)

Tx:

Dwarfism: Growth hormone deficiency

Sx:

PE:

Dx:

Tx:

Prolactinoma:

Sx: Breast enlargement, amenorrhea, decreased libido

PE:

Dx:

Tx:

Hyperprolactinemia: **Most common cause is prolactinoma**

Increased prolactin levels inhibit gonadotropin releasing hormone which causes a decrease in FSH/LH

Sx:

PE:

Dx:

Tx:

Hypogonadism:

Sx:

PE:

Dx: Low testosterone

Tx:

Pituitary Adenoma:

Sx:

PE:

Dx: Pituitary MRI

Tx:

Diabetes Mellitus

Insulin = hormone secreted by pancreatic B cells (allows glucose into cells)

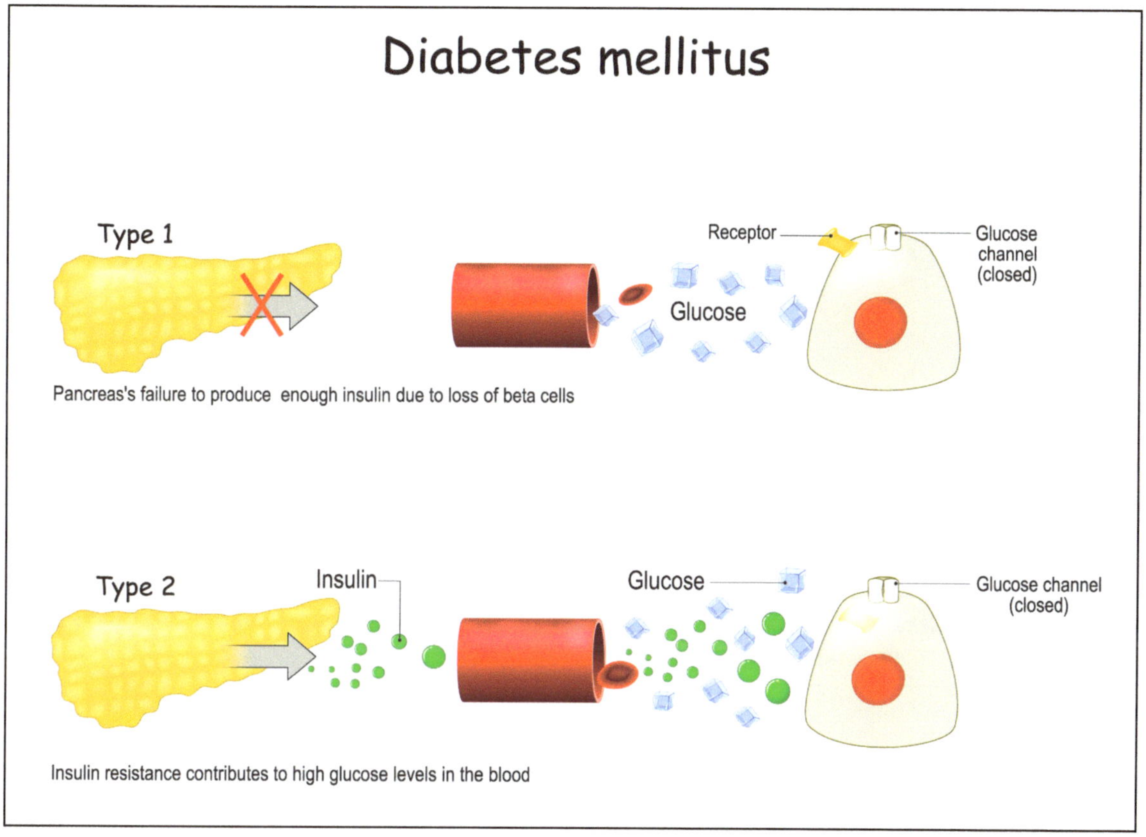

Diabetes Mellitus I: Autoimmune

Sx: Polyuria, polydipsia, polyphagia

PE:

Dx:

Tx:

Diabetes Mellitus II:

Sx:

PE:

Dx: Hb A1C > 6.5%, fasting glucose > 125 mg/dL, random glucose > 200 mg/dL

Tx:

Diabetic Ketoacidosis (DKA): Complication often associated with type I diabetes

Sx:

PE: Fruity breath

Dx:

Tx:

Hyperosmolar Hyperglycemic Syndrome (HHS): Complication of type II diabetes

Sx:

PE:

Dx: Hyperglycemia (glucose > 600mg/dL) and hyperosmolality (> 320 mOsm/kg)

Tx:

Hypoglycemia:

Sx: Nausea, confusion, sweating, palpitations, hunger

PE:

Dx:

Tx:

Metabolic Syndrome (Including Insulin Resistance):

Sx: Skin tags, acanthosis nigricans, central abdominal obesity

PE:

Dx:

Tx:

Gynecomastia:

Sx: Enlargement of breast tissue

PE:

Dx:

Tx:

Multiple Endocrine Neoplasia (MEN): **Hereditary tumor syndromes with distinct patterns of organ involvement**

Sx:

PE:

Dx:

Tx:

Diabetes Medications

Insulin:

MOA = ____________________

Indication(s) = ____________________

Side Effects = ____________________

Types/ Examples = ____________________

Biguanides - Metformin:

MOA = ____________________

Indication(s) = ____________________

Side Effects = ____________________

Types/ Examples = ____________________

Sulfonylureas:

MOA = ____________________

Indication(s) = ____________________

Side Effects = ____________________

Types/ Examples = ____________________

Meglitinides:

MOA = ____________________

Indication(s) = ____________________

Side Effects = ____________________

Types/ Examples = ____________________

Thiazolidinediones:

MOA = ____________________

Indication(s) = ____________________

Side Effects = ____________________

Types/ Examples = ____________________

Alpha - Glucosidase Inhibitor:

MOA = ____________________

Indication(s) = ____________________

Side Effects = ____________________

Types/ Examples = ____________________

GLP - 1 Agonists:

MOA = ____________________

Indication(s) = ____________________

Side Effects = ____________________

Types/ Examples = ____________________

DDP - 4 Antagonists:

MOA = ____________________

Indication(s) = ____________________

Side Effects = ____________________

Types/ Examples = ____________________

Medications

______________: MOA = ______________________________

Indication(s)=______________________________

Side Effects = ______________________________

Types/ Examples = ______________________________

____

____

______________: MOA = ______________________________

Indication(s)=______________________________

Side Effects = ______________________________

Types/ Examples = ______________________________

____

____

______________: MOA = ______________________________

Indication(s)=______________________________

Side Effects = ______________________________

Types/ Examples = ______________________________

____

____

______________: MOA = ______________________________

Indication(s)=______________________________

Side Effects = ______________________________

Types/ Examples = ______________________________

____

____

______________: MOA = ______________________________

Indication(s)=______________________________

Side Effects = ______________________________

Types/ Examples = ______________________________

____

____

Medications

____________________: MOA = ____

Indication(s)=____

Side Effects = ____

Types/ Examples = ____

____

____

____________________: MOA = ____

Indication(s)=____

Side Effects = ____

Types/ Examples = ____

____

____

____________________: MOA = ____

Indication(s)=____

Side Effects = ____

Types/ Examples = ____

____

____

____________________: MOA = ____

Indication(s)=____

Side Effects = ____

Types/ Examples = ____

____

____

____________________: MOA = ____

Indication(s)=____

Side Effects = ____

Types/ Examples = ____

____

____

Psychiatric

Depressive Disorders

Major Depressive Disorder: SIEGCAPS > 2 weeks

Sx:

PE:

Dx: DSM V

Tx:

Persistent Depressive Disorder (PDD) "Dysthymia": Symptoms > 2 years with no more than 2 months no symptoms

Sx:

PE:

Dx: DSM V

Tx:

Premenstrual Dysphoric Disorder (PMDD): Symptoms occurring 1-2 weeks before menses (luteal phase), relieved within 2-3 days of the onset of menses + 7 days no symptoms during follicular phase

Sx: Irritability, labile mood, anger

PE:

Dx: DSM V

Tx:

Seasonal Affect Disorder (SAD): **Winter months, less sunlight**

Sx: Persistent low mood, anhedonia, low energy

PE:

Dx: DSM V

Tx:

Adjustment Disorder: **Symptoms of emotion and behavior occurring within 3 months of a stressor**

Sx: Impairment of functioning

PE:

Dx: DSM V

Tx:

Bipolar Disorders

Bipolar I: **At least 1 manic episode with or without depression, must have 1 manic episode lasting > 1 week**

Sx: DIGFAST

PE:

Dx: DSM V

____________________________ Tx:

____

____

Bipolar II: **Major depressive disorder + 1 or more episode(s) of hypomania lasting 4-6 days**

Sx:

PE:

Dx: DSM V

____________________________ Tx:

____

____

Cyclothymic Disorder: **At least 2 years of hypomanic and depressive episodes that do not meet criteria for Bipolar I or Major Depressive Disorder**

Sx:

PE:

Dx: DSM V

____________________________ Tx:

____

____

Anxiety Disorders

Generalized Anxiety Disorder (GAD): Anxiety symptoms for 6+ months

Sx: Restlessness, Irritability, sleep disturbance

PE:

Dx: DSM V

Tx:

Panic Attack: Sense of impending doom

Sx:

PE:

Dx: DSM V

Tx:

Panic Disorder: 2+ panic attacks followed by > 1 month of worry about recurrence

Sx: Anxiety, palpitations

PE:

Dx: DSM V

Tx:

Specific Phobia: > 6 months

Sx: Persistent anxiety or fear of a specific situation or thing

PE:

Dx: DSM V

Tx:

Social Anxiety Disorder: > 6 months

Sx: Intense, persistent fear of social situations or performance

PE:

Dx: DSM V

Tx:

Agoraphobia: Fear of enclosed spaces, crowds, or leaving one's home > 6 months

Sx:

PE:

Dx: DSM V

Tx:

Obsessive Compulsive Disorder: **> 1 hour per day**

Sx: Obsessions: Intrusive, recurrent thoughts that cause anxiety or stress
Compulsions: Repetitive behaviors or mental acts to relieve anxiety

PE:

Dx: DSM V

____________________ **Tx:**

____

____

Post-Traumatic Stress Disorder (PTSD): **Trauma exposure, flashbacks > 1 month**

Sx: Nightmares, flashbacks, sleep problems, hypervigilance, avoidance of thoughts, feelings, & memories

PE:

Dx: DSM V

____________________ **Tx:**

____

____

Acute Stress Disorder: **Same as PTSD, but shorter time frame < 1 month**

Sx:

PE:

Dx: DSM V

____________________ **Tx:**

____

____

Trichotillomania: **Hair pulling disorder**

Sx: Pulling out of one's hair with repeated attempts to decrease or stop hair pulling

PE:

Dx: DSM V

Tx:

Hoarding Disorder:

Sx: Difficulty parting with possessions that congest and clutter active living areas

PE:

Dx: DSM V

Tx:

Psychotic Disorders

Delusional Disorder: > 1 month with 1 or more delusions without significant impairment in functioning

Sx: 1 or more delusions

PE:

Dx: DSM V

______________________________ Tx:

____

____

Schizophrenia: 2 or more positive symptoms > 6 months

Positive Sx: Hallucinations, delusions, or disorganized speech
Negative Sx: Blunted affect, anhedonia

PE:

Dx: DSM V

______________________________ Tx:

____

____

Brief Psychotic Disorder: Psychotic symptoms for 1 day to 1 month

Sx: Psychotic symptoms

PE:

Dx: DSM V

______________________________ Tx:

____

____

Schizophreniform: 1 month - 6 months

Sx: Same as schizophrenia

PE:

Dx: DSM V

____

____

____

Tx:

Schizoaffective Disorder:

Sx: Schizophrenia symptoms + mood symptoms

PE:

Dx: DSM V

____

____

____

Tx:

Personality Disorders
Cluster A (The Weird)

Paranoid: **Suspicious and distrusting of others**

Sx: Suspects others are exploiting them

PE:

Dx: DSM V

____

____

____

Tx:

Schizoid: **Detachment from social relationships**

Sx: No desire for close relationships

PE:

Dx: DSM V

____

____

____

Tx:

Schizotypal:

Sx: Odd beliefs or magical thinking

PE:

Dx: DSM V

____

____

____

Tx:

Cluster B (The Wild)

Antisocial: > 18 years old, behaviors deviate from societal norms, values, and laws

Sx: Non-conforming to social norms, irritable, irresponsible, lack of remorse

PE:

Dx: DSM V

____

____

____

Tx:

Histrionic: Begins early adulthood, variety of settings

Sx: Emotional, dramatic, attention seeking

PE:

Dx: DSM V

____

____

____

Tx:

Borderline:

Sx: Unstable relationships, impulsive, mood swings, recurrent suicidal behaviors, gestures or threats

PE:

Dx: DSM V

____

____

____

Tx:

Narcissistic:

Sx: Big ego, no empathy, sensitive to failure, exploit others, grandiose sense of self-importance

PE:

Dx: DSM V

____

____

____

Tx:

Cluster C (The Worried)

Avoidant:

Sx: Afraid of rejection, social inhibition

PE:

Dx: DSM V

____

____

____

Tx:

Dependent:

Sx: Afraid of abandonment, passive, low self-esteem, submissive and clingy behaviors

PE:

Dx: DSM V

____

____

____

Tx:

Obsessive Compulsive Personality Disorder:

Sx: Control, rigid, perfectionistic, expects others to meet increased standards

PE:

Dx: DSM V

____

____

____

Tx:

Somatic Disorders

Somatic Symptom Disorder: 1 or more somatic symptoms + anxiety with NO CAUSE > 6 months

Sx: High levels of anxiety about one's health

PE:

Dx: DSM V

______________________________ Tx:

____

____

Illness Anxiety Disorder: Hypochondriac with anxiety about health > 6 months

Sx:

PE:

Dx: DSM V

______________________________ Tx:

____

____

Conversion Disorder: Neuro symptoms without having a neuro or medical condition. Negative EEG and labs

Sx: Intermittent paralysis, bizarre movements

PE:

Dx: DSM V

______________________________ Tx:

____

____

Factitious Disorder: **Consciously has false symptoms to play sick role**

Sx: Person presents themselves as injured or ill

PE:

Dx: DSM V

Tx:

Factitious Disorder by Proxy: **Consciously puts false symptoms onto others**

Sx: Perpetrator, presents victim (most often their child) as injured or ill

PE:

Dx: DSM V

Tx:

Malingering: **Intentional false symptoms for external gain**

Sx: Exaggeration or fabrication of mental or physical symptoms for gain

PE:

Dx: DSM V

Tx:

Pseudocyesis: **False belief that one is pregnant**

Sx:

PE:

Dx: DSM V

Tx:

Developmental Psych and Behavioral Disorders

Attention Deficit Hyperactivity Disorder (ADHD):

Sx: Difficulty paying attention, impulsivity, and hyperactivity

PE:

Dx: DSM V

Tx:

Inattention:

Hyperactivity and Impulsivity:

Combined Type:

Autism Spectrum Disorder (ASD): Spectrum of developmental disorders

Sx: Social interaction problems, impaired communication, restricted, repetitive patterns of behavior, interests or activities

PE:

Dx: DSM V

Tx:

Conduct Disorder: < 18 years old, may progress to antisocial personality disorder

Sx: Violates rights of others, may hurt animals, lacks remorse

PE:

Dx: DSM V

Tx:

Oppositional Defiant Disorder (ODD):

Sx: Easily annoyed, often angry, spiteful, deliberately annoys

PE:

Dx: DSM V

Tx:

Disruptive Mood Dysregulation Disorder:

Sx: Temper outburst, out of proportion to situation or provoking event, irritable mood between outbursts

PE:

Dx: DSM V

Tx:

Eating Disorders

Anorexia Nervosa: Preoccupation with body weight & image

Restrictive type Sx:

Dx: DSM V

Binge eating and purging type Sx:

Dx: DSM V

Tx:

Bulimia Nervosa: Binging and inappropriate compensatory behaviors (usually purging)

Sx:

PE: Russell's sign

Dx: DSM V

Tx:

Binge Eating Disorder: **Recurrent episodes of binge eating - at least weekly for 3 months**

Sx:

PE:

Dx: DSM V

____

____

____

Tx:

Body Dysmorphia:

Sx: Preoccupation with defects or flaws in one's personal appearance

PE:

Dx: DSM V

____

____

____

Tx:

Sleep Disorders

Narcolepsy: Episodes occurring at least 3 times per week for 3+ months

Sx: Chronic daytime sleepiness, cataplexy

PE:

Dx: DSM V

Tx:

Hypersomnolence: Excessive sleepiness

Sx: Prolonged sleep episodes longer than 9 hours per day

PE:

Dx: DSM V

Tx:

Insomnia:

Sx: Difficulty initiating sleep, difficulty maintaining sleep, waking up early

PE:

Dx: DSM V

Tx:

Nightmare Disorders:

Sx:

PE:

Dx: DSM V

Tx:

Parasomnias

Sleepwalking:

Sx: Walking around while sleeping

PE:

Dx: DSM V

Tx:

Sleep Terrors:

Sx: Abrupt arousal from sleep, sometimes with panic and screaming

PE:

Dx: DSM V

Tx:

Drug Abuse/Dependence

Tobacco Use Dependance:

Sx:

PE:

Dx: DSM V

Tx:

Nicotine withdrawal:

Sx:

Alcohol Use/Dependance:

Sx: Increased CNS activity, seizures, hallucinations, delirium tremens

PE:

Dx: DSM V

Tx:

Alcohol withdrawal:

Sx:

Opioid Use/Dependance:

Sx: Pupillary constriction, altered mental status, respiratory depression

PE:

Dx: DSM V

Tx:

____

____

____

Opioid withdrawal:

Sx:

Cocaine Intoxication:

Sx: Tremor, flushing, hyperthermia, pupillary dilation, cold sweats

PE:

Dx: DSM V

Tx:

____

____

____

Cocaine withdrawal:

Sx:

PCP Intoxication:

Sx: Impulsivity, fear, rage, psychosis, delirium, hallucinations

PE:

Dx: DSM V

Tx:

PCP withdrawal

Sx:

Marijuana Intoxication:

Sx: Euphoria, giddiness, anxiety, disinhibition, intensification of sensory experiences, cotton mouth

PE:

Dx: DSM V

Tx:

Marijuana withdrawal:

Sx:

Dissociative Disorders

Dissociative Identity Disorder (DID):

Sx: 2+ distinct personality states

PE:

Dx: DSM V

Tx:

Dissociative Amnesia:

Sx: Difficulty recalling autobiographical information, usually related to trauma or stress

PE:

Dx: DSM V

Tx:

Dissociative Fugue:

Sx: Amnesia + travel

PE:

Dx: DSM V

Tx:

Depersonalization/Derealization Disorder:

Sx: Unreality, detachment, feeling like an outside observer

PE:

Dx: DMS V

Tx:

Types of Abuse

Child Physical Abuse: Non-accidental physical injury to a child

Sx: Bruising, fractures, death

PE:

Dx: DSM V

Tx:

Child Neglect:

Sx: Deprivation of age-appropriate needs resulting in physical or psychological harm

PE:

Dx: DSM V

Tx:

Sexual Abuse:

Sx:

PE:

Dx: DSM V

Tx:

Intimate Partner Abuse:

Sx:

PE:

Dx: DSM V

Tx:

Sexual Disorders

Exhibitionistic Disorder:

Sx: Sexual arousal from exposing oneself

PE:

Dx: DSM V

Tx:

Fetishistic Disorder:

Sx: Sexual arousal from nonliving objects or nongenital body parts

PE:

Dx: DSM V

Tx:

Frotteuristic Disorder:

Sx: Sexual arousal from touching or rubbing up against a non-consenting person

PE:

Dx: DSM V

Tx:

Pedophile Disorder:

Sx: Sexual fantasies, urges involving prepubescent child or children

PE:

Dx: DSM V

Tx:

Sexual Masochism Disorder:

Sx: Sexual arousal in response to pain or humiliation

PE:

Dx: DSM V

Tx:

Sexual Sadism Disorder:

Sx: Sexual arousal from the physical or psychological suffering of another person

PE:

Dx: DSM V

Tx:

Voyeuristic Disorder:

Sx: Sexual arousal from watching naked, unsuspecting persons

PE:

Dx: DSM V

Tx:

Misc. Psych Disorders

Grief Reaction: Severe symptoms > 1 year

Sx:

PE:

Dx:

Tx:

Suicide:

Sx:

PE:

Dx:

Tx:

Serotonin Syndrome: Life threatening, increased serotonin within 6-24 hours of initiation or change in serotonergic drugs

Sx:

PE:

Dx:

Tx:

Neuroleptic Malignant Syndrome: **Life threatening, complication of treatment with antipsychotics**

Sx: Hyperthermia, altered mental status

PE:

Dx:

____

____

____

Tx:

Tourette Syndrome:

Sx: "Tics" repeated sounds, movements, or twitches

PE:

Dx:

____

____

____

Tx:

Postpartum Depression: ***In Women's Health***

Medications

______________: MOA = ______________
Indication(s)=______________
Side Effects = ______________
Types/ Examples = ______________

______________: MOA = ______________
Indication(s)=______________
Side Effects = ______________
Types/ Examples = ______________

______________: MOA = ______________
Indication(s)=______________
Side Effects = ______________
Types/ Examples = ______________

______________: MOA = ______________
Indication(s)=______________
Side Effects = ______________
Types/ Examples = ______________

______________: MOA = ______________
Indication(s)=______________
Side Effects = ______________
Types/ Examples = ______________

Medications

______________: MOA = ______________

Indication(s)=______________

Side Effects = ______________

Types/ Examples = ______________

____

____

______________: MOA = ______________

Indication(s)=______________

Side Effects = ______________

Types/ Examples = ______________

____

____

______________: MOA = ______________

Indication(s)=______________

Side Effects = ______________

Types/ Examples = ______________

____

____

______________: MOA = ______________

Indication(s)=______________

Side Effects = ______________

Types/ Examples = ______________

____

____

______________: MOA = ______________

Indication(s)=______________

Side Effects = ______________

Types/ Examples = ______________

____

____

Women's Health

Menstruation Disorders

Amenorrhea: **Transient or permanent absence of menstrual flow**

Primary amenorrhea:

Sx: No menses by age 15

PE:

Dx:

______________________________________ **Tx:**

____

____

Causes: Hypothalamic, pituitary insufficiency, low FSH & LH, anorexia

---

Turner Syndrome: **XO karyotype**

Sx:

PE: Webbed neck, broad chest

Dx: High FSH

______________________________________ **Tx:**

____

____

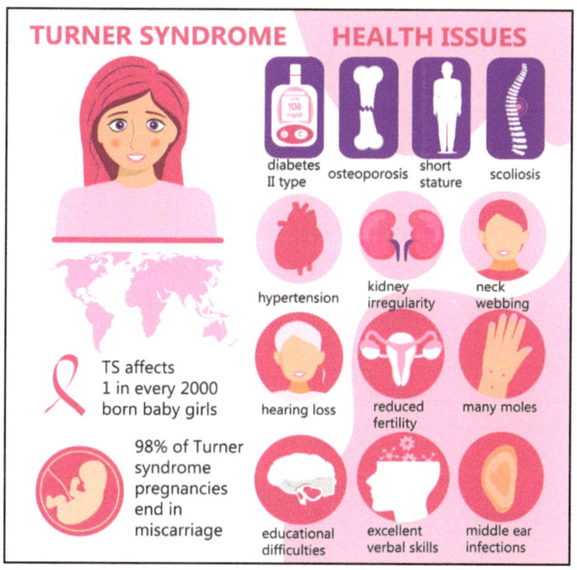

Androgen Insensitivity:

Sx:

PE: Breast development only

Dx: High testosterone

Tx:

Müllerian Agenesis:

Sx:

PE: Secondary sex characteristics, no uterus

Dx:

Tx:

Imperforate Hymen: Blocked vaginal opening

Sx: Can block menstrual flow

PE:

Dx:

Tx:

Secondary Amenorrhea:

Sx: Absence of menses for 3+ cycles after previously having normal periods

PE:

Dx:

Tx:

Causes: Hypothyroid, prolactinoma

Asherman Syndrome: Amenorrhea after an intrauterine procedure (e.g., D&C, or complication from procedural surgery)

Sx:

PE: No specific findings

Dx:

Tx:

Dysfunctional Uterine Bleeding

Polymenorrhagia: Menses < 21 days

Tx:

Menorrhagia: Prolonged bleeding (> 7 days or > 80 mL) during menses

Tx:

Metrorrhagia: Uterine bleeding that occurs more frequently and irregularly between menses

Tx:

Menometrorrhagia: Increased blood loss during menses as well as frequent and irregular bleeding between menses

Tx:

Oligomenorrhea: Long intervals between menses > 35 days

Tx:

Dx:

Painful Uterine Bleeding

Dysmenorrhea: Pain peaks 24 hours after the onset of menses and subsides after 2-3 days

Tx:

Primary Dysmenorrhea: No organic cause - excessive prostaglandins

Tx:

Secondary Dysmenorrhea: Painful menstruation caused by clinically identifiable cause

Etiology: Endometriosis, adenomyosis, polyps, fibroids, PID, IUD, adhesions, tumors

Tx:

Dx:

Menstruation

Follicular (Proliferative) Phase: Days 0-14: Estrogen prominent

GnRH (from hypothalamus) stimulates FSH and LH (from anterior pituitary) which then triggers ovulation

Ovulation:

GnRH (from hypothalamus) stimulates FSH and LH (from anterior pituitary) which then triggers ovulation

Luteal (Secretory) Phase: Days 15-28: Progesterone prominent

After ovulation, the follicle becomes the corpus luteum, which secretes progesterone and provides negative feedback to FSH & LH

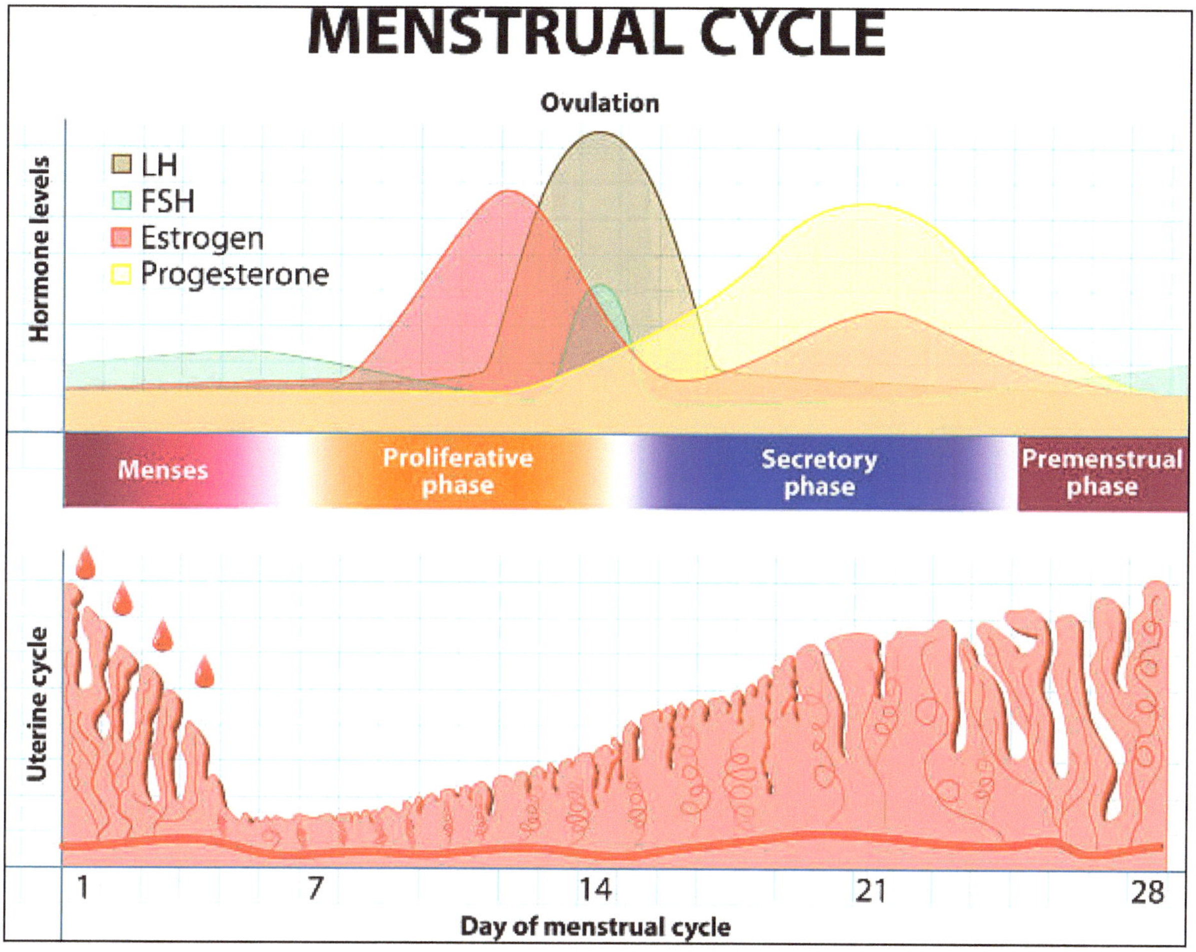
MENSTRUAL CYCLE
Ovulation
LH
FSH
Estrogen
Progesterone
Hormone levels
Menses
Proliferative phase
Secretory phase
Premenstrual phase
Uterine cycle
1
7
14
21
28
Day of menstrual cycle

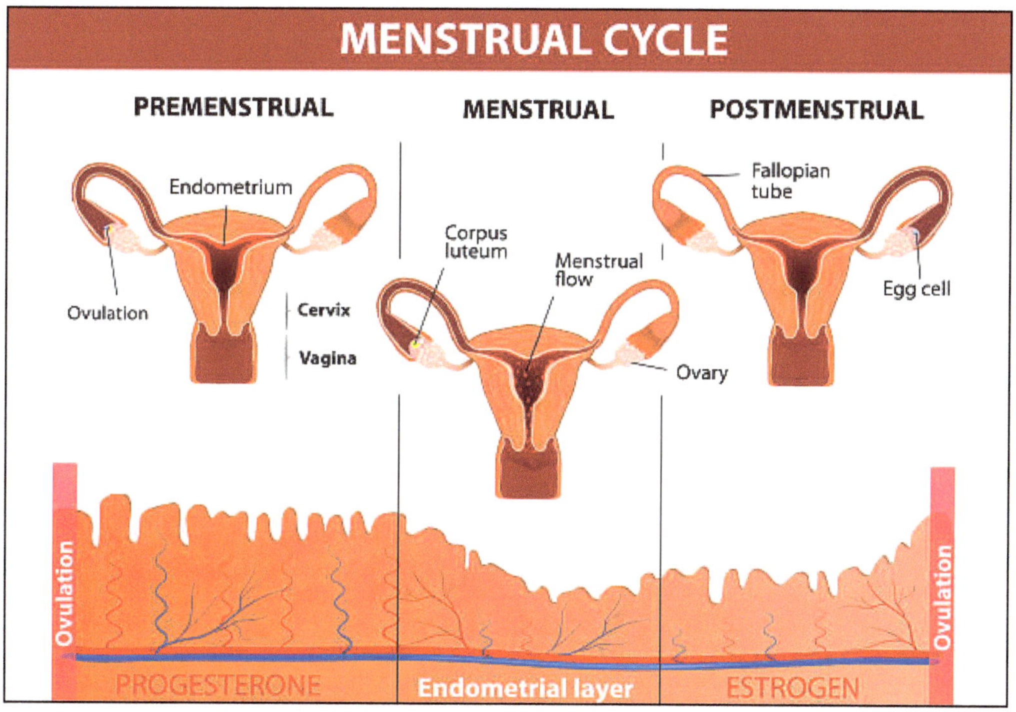
MENSTRUAL CYCLE
PREMENSTRUAL
MENSTRUAL
POSTMENSTRUAL
Endometrium
Ovulation
Cervix
Vagina
Corpus luteum
Menstrual flow
Ovary
Fallopian tube
Egg cell
Ovulation
PROGESTERONE
Endometrial layer
ESTROGEN
Ovulation

Premenstrual Syndrome (PMS):

Sx: Bloating & irritability during luteal phase

PE:

Dx:

Tx:

Menopause: 12 or more months of amenorrhea

Sx: Hot flashes, night sweats, irritability, vaginal dryness

PE:

Dx: Labs: Increased FSH, decreased estradiol

Tx:

Atrophic Vaginitis: Pale, atrophic epithelium with flattened rugae

Sx: Vaginal dryness, burning, possible dysuria

PE:

Dx:

Tx:

Birth Control

Hormonal IUD:

MOA = ______________________________

Indication(s)=______________________________

Side Effects=______________________________

Types/ Examples=______________________________

Non-Hormonal IUD:

MOA = ______________________________

Indication(s)=______________________________

Side Effects=______________________________

Types/ Examples=______________________________

Nexplanon:

MOA = ______________________________

Indication(s)=______________________________

Side Effects=______________________________

Types/ Examples=______________________________

Depo-Provera:

MOA = ______________________________

Indication(s)=______________________________

Side Effects=______________________________

Types/ Examples=______________________________

Vaginal Ring:

MOA = ______________________________

Indication(s)=______________________________

Side Effects=______________________________

Types/ Examples=______________________________

Transdermal Patch:

MOA = ____________________

Indication(s)= ____________________

Side Effects= ____________________

Types/ Examples= ____________________

Combined Oral Contraception:

MOA = ____________________

Indication(s)= ____________________

Side Effects= ____________________

Types/ Examples= ____________________

Progesterone Only Pill:

MOA = ____________________

Indication(s)= ____________________

Side Effects= ____________________

Types/ Examples= ____________________

Emergency Contraception:

MOA = ____________________

Indication(s)= ____________________

Side Effects= ____________________

Types/ Examples= ____________________

Breast Disorders

Mastitis: S. aureus

Sx: Unilateral breast pain, tenderness, warmth, swelling

PE: Cracked nipples and fissures

Dx:

Tx:

Breast Abscess: S. aureus

Sx: Red, mass, pain, fluctuance, induration

PE:

Dx:

Tx:

Fibrocystic Breast Changes: Typically presents prior to menstruation

Sx:

PE:

Dx:

Tx:

Fibroadenoma: **Common benign solid tumor**

Sx: Round, firm, discrete, mobile, non-tender mass

PE:

Dx:

Tx:

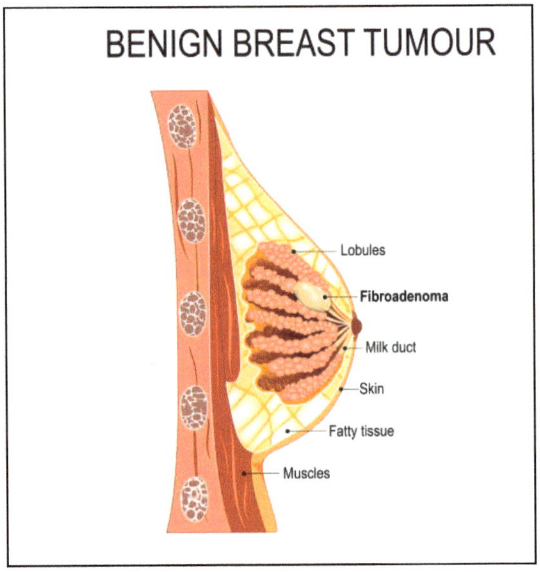

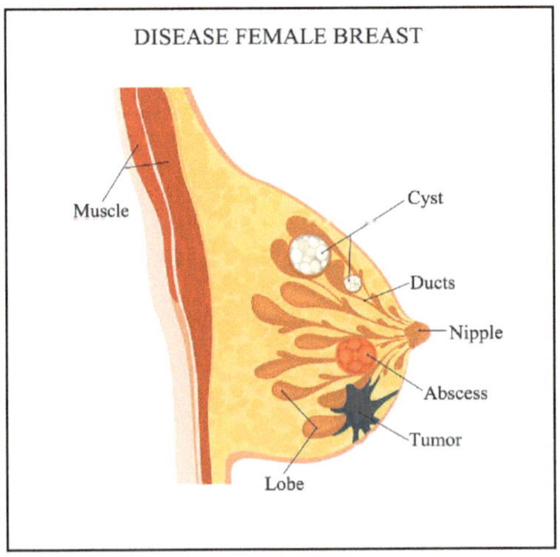

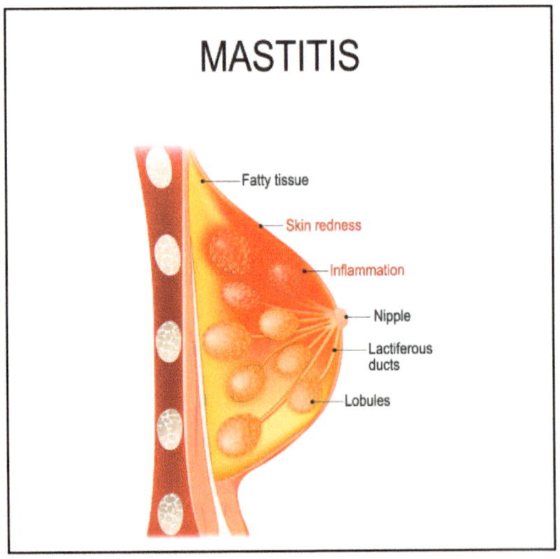

Breast Cancer

Invasive Ductal Carcinoma:

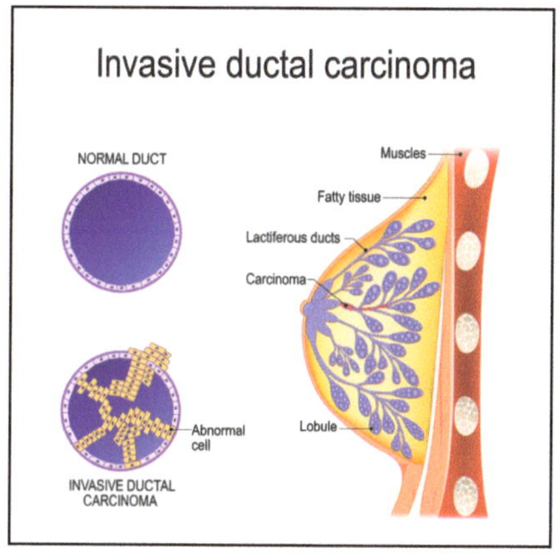

Sx: Can be asymptomatic

PE:

Dx: Mammogram

Tx:

Invasive Lobular Carcinoma: Most common type

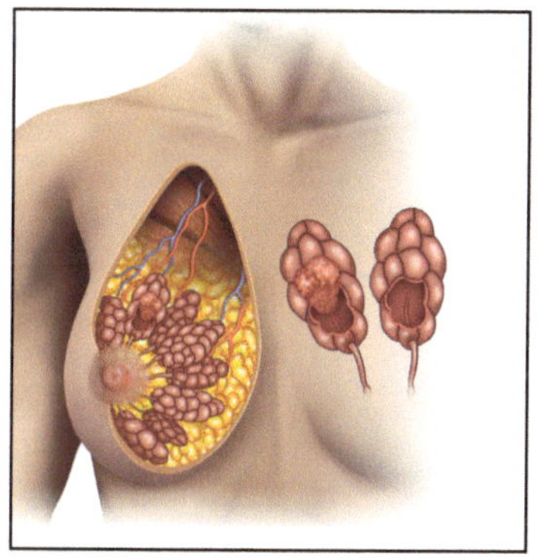

Sx: Can be asymptomatic

PE:

Dx: Mammogram

Tx:

Paget's Disease of the Breast:

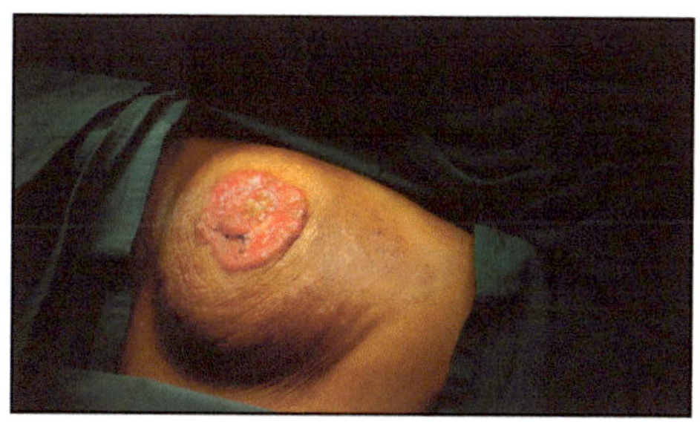

Sx: Itchy, scaling rash on the nipples & areola

PE:

Dx:

Tx:

Breast Cancer Screening and Prevention:

Other GYN Dysplasias & Carcinomas

Cervical Dysplasia:

Sx:

PE:

Dx: Pap smear

- ASC - US
- LSIL - low grade (CIN I)
- ASC - H
- HSIL - high grade (CIN II, III)

____

____

____

Tx:

Cervical Cancer:

Risk Factors: Human papilloma virus (HPV) **in Infectious Disease*, smoking

Sx: Post-coital bleeding or spotting

PE:

Dx: Pap smear

- ASC - US
- LSIL
- HSIL

____

____

____

Tx:

Cervical Cancer Screening:

HPV vaccination:

Endometrial Hyperplasia:

Risk Factors: Prolonged unopposed estrogen, chronic anovulation, obesity, PCOS, Tamoxifen use

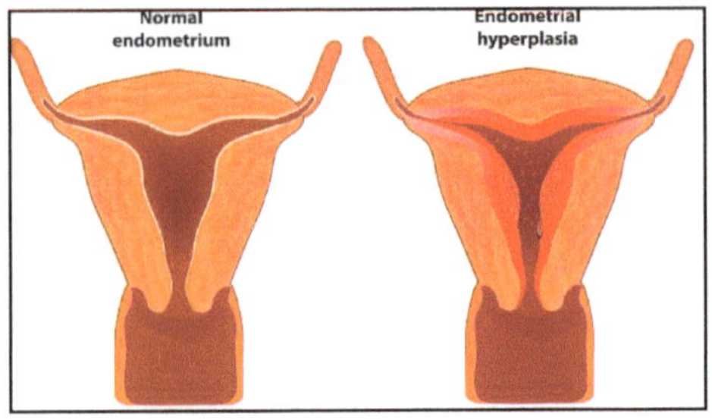

Sx: Abnormal uterine bleeding

PE:

Dx:

____

____

____

Tx:

Endometrial Cancer: Most common GYN malignancy

Risk Factors: Endometrial hyperplasia, high estrogen exposure, obesity, PCOS

Sx: Postmenopausal bleeding

PE:

Dx:

____

____

____

Tx:

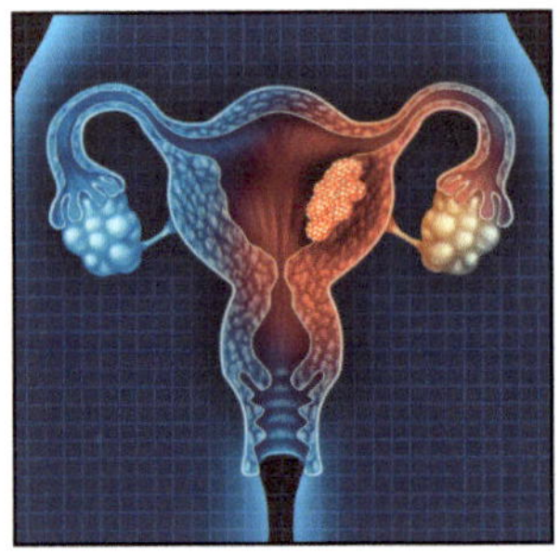

Ovarian Cancer: Epithelial carcinoma is most common

Risk Factors: Nulligravida, early menarche, late menopause, endometriosis

Early Sx:

Late Sx:

PE: Adnexal mass, abdominal bloating

Dx:

____

____

____

Tx:

Protective Factors: OCP use, breastfeeding

Vaginal Cancer: RARE

Risk Factors: Smoking, HPV, multiple partners, Diethylstilbestrol (DES)

Sx: Postmenopausal & postcoital bleeding

PE: Vaginal mass

Dx:

Tx:

Vulvar Cancer:

Sx: Vaginal pruritus

PE: Red, white ulcerative, or raised crusted lesion

Dx:

Tx:

Postmenopausal Bleeding:

Sx: Vaginal bleeding occurring after menopause

PE:

Dx:

Tx:

Female Reproductive Organ Concerns

Polycystic Ovarian Syndrome (PCOS):

Sx: Amenorrhea, obesity, hirsutism, polycystic ovaries, increased LH & FSH, androgen excess

PE:

Dx:

Tx:

Ovarian Cyst: Most common are follicular cyst

Sx: Pelvic pain, bloating

PE: Palpable abdominal mass

Dx:

Tx:

Ovarian Cyst Rupture:

Sx: Sudden abdominal pain, fever, vomiting

PE:

Dx:

Tx:

Ovarian Torsion: EMERGENCY!!!

Sx: Waxing and waning pain, N/V/D, sudden, sharp, unilateral pain

PE:

Dx: Transvaginal US

Tx:

Endometriosis:

Sx: Dyspareunia, dyschezia, dysmenorrhea

PE: Uterus is fixed and retroflexed

Dx:

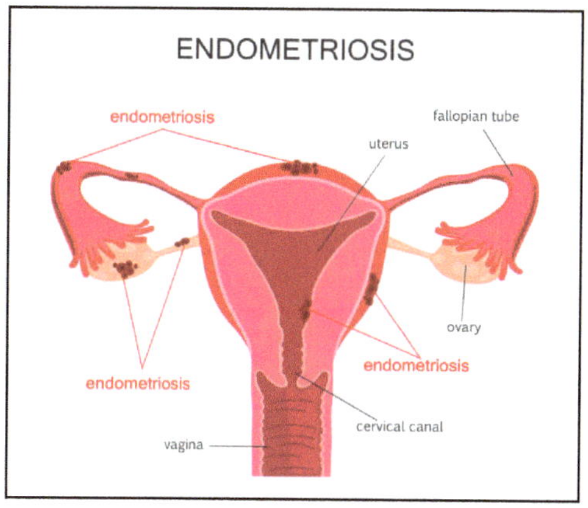

Tx:

Chronic Endometriosis:

Sx: Abdominal swelling, abnormal vaginal bleeding

PE:

Dx:

Tx:

Leiomyoma: Uterine fibroids

Sx:

PE:

Dx: US and/or MRI

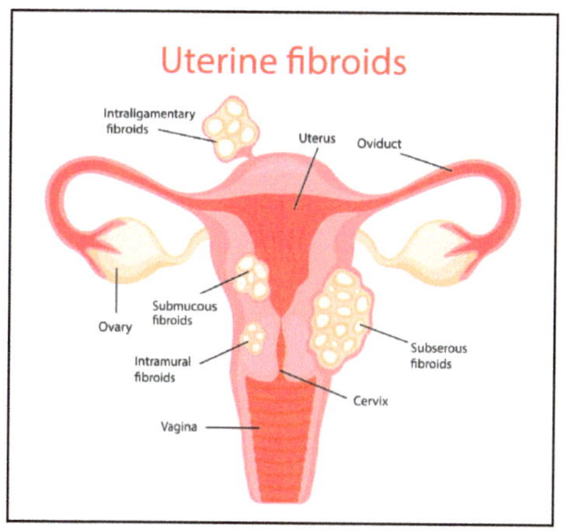

Tx:

Adenomyoma:

Sx: Cramping, metrorrhagia, dysmenorrhea

PE:

Dx:

Tx:

Bartholin Cyst & Abscess:

Sx: Vulvar pain and/or mass

PE:

Dx:

Tx:

Toxic Shock Syndrome:

Sx: Rapid onset fever, body aches, headache, chills

PE:

Dx:

Tx:

Misc. Women's Health

Bladder Prolapse (Cystocele): **Anterior vagina**

Sx: Vaginal fullness "heaviness", urinary urgency & frequency

PE:

Dx:

____

____

____

Tx:

Rectal Prolapse (Rectocele): **Posterior wall**

Sx:

PE:

Dx:

____

____

____

Tx:

Uterine Prolapse: **Uterine herniation into the vagina**

Sx: Vaginal protrusion & pressure

PE:

Dx:

____

____

____

Tx:

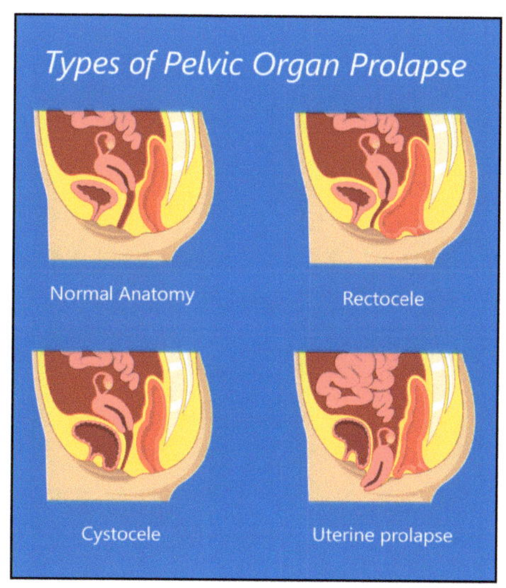

Uncomplicated Pregnancy

Hormones

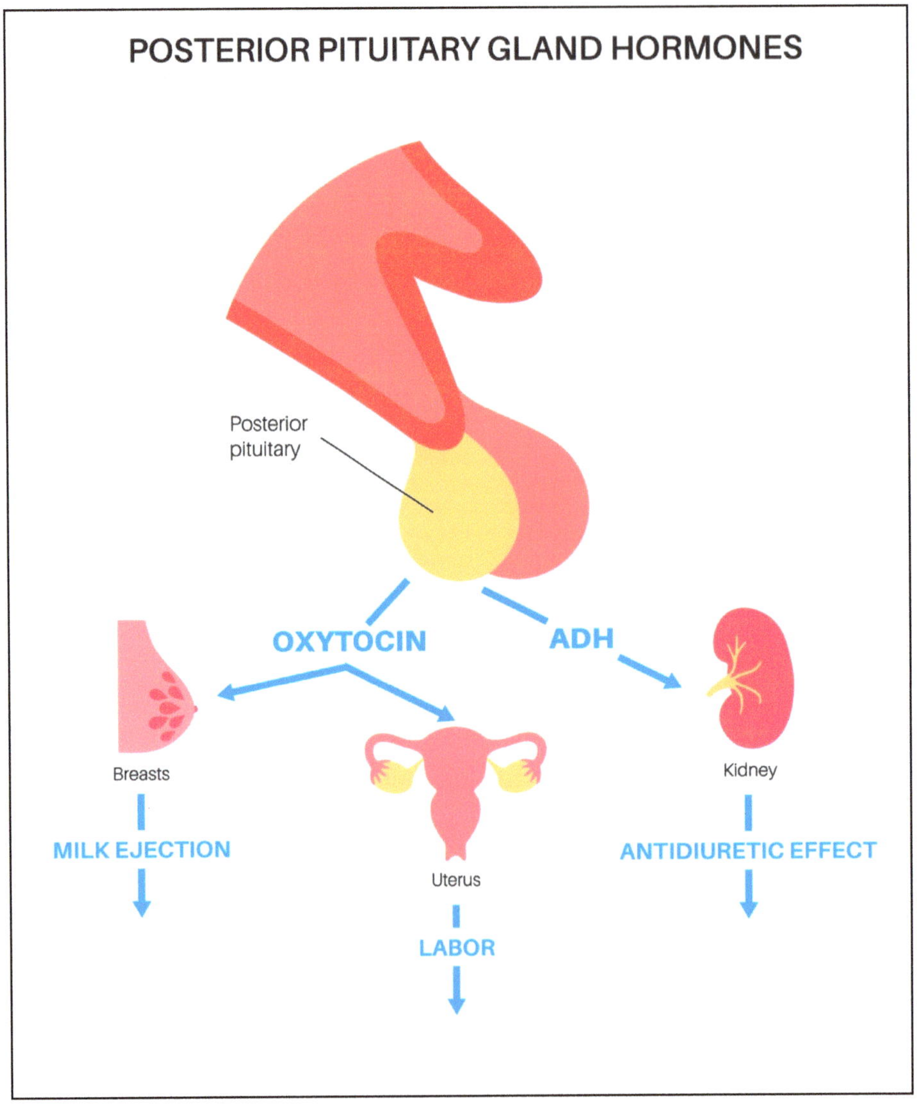

Trimesters

1st Trimester: Weeks 1-12

Fetal heart tones by 12 weeks

Chronic villus sampling 10-12 weeks

2nd Trimester: Weeks 13-27

15-18 weeks = amniocentesis

24 weeks = 1 hour glucose challenge test

3rd Trimester: Weeks 28-40

28-30 weeks = Rhogam injection if Rh negative

35-37 = group B strep

36-40 = gonorrhea & chlamydia cultures

UA & blood glucose

Pregnancy Terms:

Hegar's sign = softening of the uterus, possible early sign of pregnancy

Goodell's sign = softening of the cervix, possible early sign of pregnancy

Chadwick's sign = increased vascularity, purplish-blue color. Possible early sign of pregnancy

Naegele's rule = 1st day of last menses + 7 days - 3 months + 1 year

Gravida: Number of times a woman has been pregnant

Parity: Number of pregnancies that led to a birth either at or after 20 weeks

T (term) = number born at 37 weeks or older

P (preterm) = born after 20 weeks but before 37 weeks

A (abortion) = all pregnancy losses prior to 20 weeks

L (living) = infant who lives beyond 30 days

Nulligravida: Woman who currently is not pregnant and never has been pregnant

Primigravida: Woman who currently is pregnant and has never been pregnant before

Multigravida: Woman who currently is pregnant and who has been pregnant before

Nullipara: Woman who has never completed a pregnancy beyond 20 weeks

Primipara: Woman who has delivered a fetus or fetuses born alive or dead with an estimate length of gestation of 20 weeks for the first time

Multipara: Woman who has delivered a fetus or fetuses born alive or dead with an estimate length of gestation of 20 weeks multiple times

Women's Health Tidbits:

Pregnancy is a hypercoagulable state

Appendectomy is the most common surgery during pregnancy

The placenta secretes estrogen, progesterone, relaxin, and hCG

Vaginal pH during pregnancy = 3.5-6.0

Pregnancy increases cardiac output, decreases blood pressure, and increases total red blood cells

Decreased hematocrit = physiologic anemia

Fundal Height:

- 12 weeks - above pubic symphysis
- 16 weeks - midway between pubis & umbilicus
- 20 weeks - umbilicus
- 38 weeks - 2-3 cm below xiphoid

Vaccines in Pregnancy:

Inactivated influenza can be given in 3rd trimester during flu season

Cannot give live attenuated vaccines (MMR, varicella)

Tdap encouraged in pregnancy, no harm to fetus, between 27 & 36 weeks

Stages of Labor

Apgar Score

Intrapartum

Pregnancy Complications

Ectopic Pregnancy: **Pregnancy outside uterine cavity - most commonly occurs in the fallopian tube**

Sx: Unilateral pelvic pain, vaginal bleeding, referred shoulder or upper abdominal pain

PE:

Dx: B-hCG > 1500

US "ring of fire"

____

____

____

Tx:

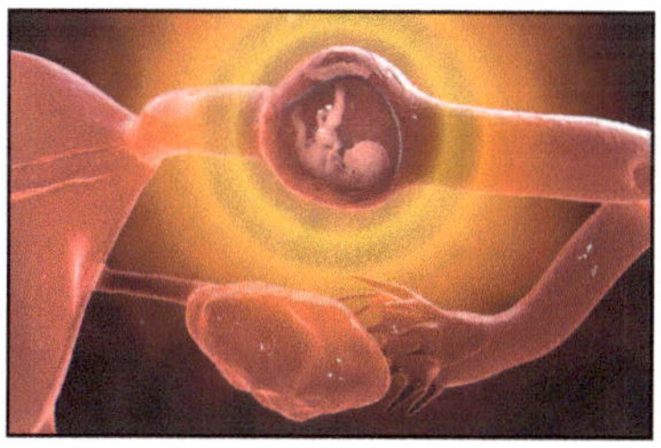

Gestational Trophoblastic Disease: **Molar pregnancy - Choriocarcinoma**

Sx: Painless vaginal bleeding

PE:

Dx: hCG higher than expected

US = "snow storm" "swiss cheese"

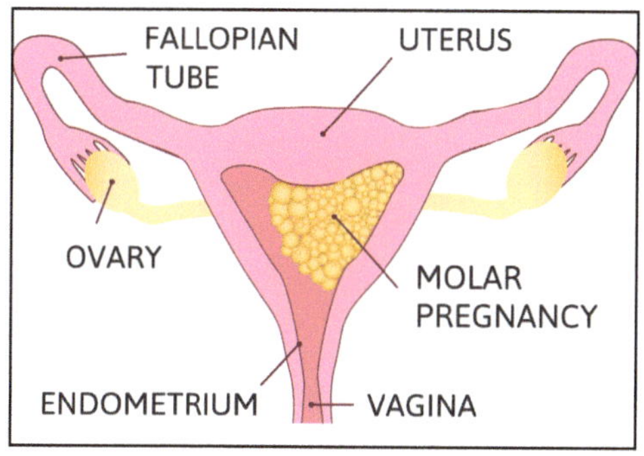

____

____

____

Tx:

Complete =

Incomplete =

Spontaneous Abortion = before 20 weeks

Threatened: Vaginal bleeding, closed cervix

Sx:

Tx:

Incomplete: Cervical os dilated with some products of conception visible < 20 weeks

Sx:

Tx:

Inevitable: Cervical os dilated without products < 20 weeks

Sx:

Tx:

Missed Abortion: Death of fetus without symptons < 20 weeks

Sx:

Tx:

Dx: US

Elective Abortion:

Sx:

PE:

Dx:

Tx:

Infertility:

Sx:

PE:

Dx: Hysterosalpingogram, semen analysis

______________________________ **Tx:**

____

____

Multiple Gestation:

Dizygotic (fraternal): Fertilization of 2 ova by 2 different sperm

Monozygotic (identical): Fertilization of 1 ovum that splits

Sx:

PE:

Dx:

______________________________ **Tx:**

____

____

Incompetent Cervix: Premature cervical shortening or dilation in the second or early third trimesters

Sx:

PE: Cervical dilation > 2 cm, painless

Dx:

______________________________ **Tx:**

____

____

Rh Factor: Babies at risk = (-Rh) mother, (+Rh) father or unknown

1st pregnancy is good, 2nd at risk

Sx:

PE:

Dx:

______________________________ **Tx:**

____

____

Preeclampsia:

Sx: Hypertension, proteinuria +/- edema after 20 weeks

Dx: Mild: 140/90 - 160/110 & proteinuria > 300 mg/24 hour or +1 dipstick

Dx: Severe: > 160/110 & proteinuria > 5g/24 hour or +3 on dipstick

Tx:

HELLP (Hemolysis, Elevated Liver Enzymes, and Low Platelets):

Sx: Abdominal pain, vision changes

PE:

Dx:

Tx:

Eclampsia: Hypertension + proteinuria + seizures or coma

Sx:

PE:

Dx: Same as Preeclampsia

Tx:

Gestational Hypertension: Symptoms after 20 weeks & resolves by 12 weeks postpartum

Sx:

PE:

Dx: BP > 150/90

Tx:

Chronic Hypertension: Symptoms before 20 weeks

Sx:

PE:

Dx: Mild: 140/90
Moderate: 150/100
Severe: 160/110

Tx:

Uterine Rupture:

Sx: Excessive vaginal bleeding, pain between contractions

PE:

Dx:

Tx:

Gestational Diabetes:

Sx:

PE:

Dx:

Test 1: 1 hour, 50g, glucose challenge test (performed between 24-28 weeks)

Test 2: If 1 hour test failed, proceed to 3 hour, 100g, glucose tolerance test.

To fail the 3 hour test there must be 2 abnormal values

Initial fasting: 95

1st hour: 180

2nd hour: 155

3rd hour: 140

Tx:

Pregestational Diabetes:

Sx:

PE:

Dx: Fasting blood glucose > 126, A1C > 6.5, random blood glucose > 200

Tx:

Preterm Labor: Labor before 37 weeks

Sx: Contractions, back ache

PE:

Dx:

Tx:

Placental Abruption: Separation of the placenta partially or totally from its implantation site before delivery

Risk Factors: Smoking, cocaine, trauma

Sx: Bleeding, abdominal PAIN

PE:

Dx: US

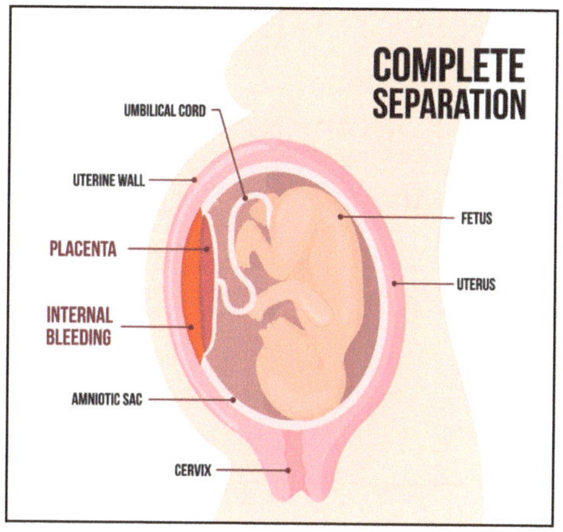

____

____

____

Tx:

Placenta Previa: Placenta that is implanted either over or near the internal cervical os

Risk Factors: Prior C-section, multiple gestation, multiple induced abortions

Sx: PAINLESS vaginal bleeding

PE:

Dx:

____

____

____

Tx:

Classifications:

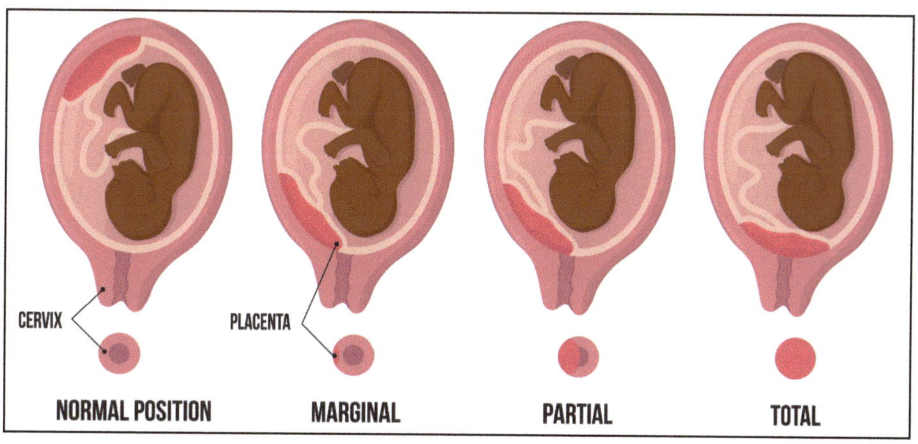

Labor & Delivery Complications

Premature Rupture Of Membranes (PROM): Rupture of amniotic sac before regular contractions start.

Preterm PROM (PROM): PROM before 37 weeks gestation

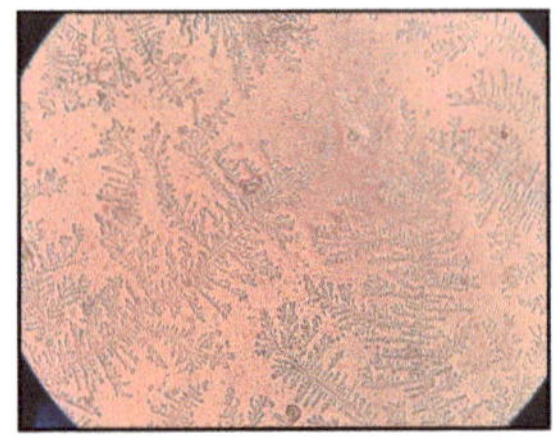

Risk Factors:

Sx:

PE:

Dx: Nitrazine paper test: Turns blue if pH >7, "ferning" on microscopy

Tx:

Placental Insufficiency: Placenta is damaged or doesn't develop appropriately

Sx:

PE:

Dx:

Tx:

Umbilical Cord Prolapse: Umbilical cord protrudes out of vagina

Sx:

PE: Bradycardia, variable decelerations

Dx:

Tx:

Breech: Presenting with buttocks and/or feet at cervix

Sx:

PE:

Dx:

______________________________ Tx:

____

____

Types:

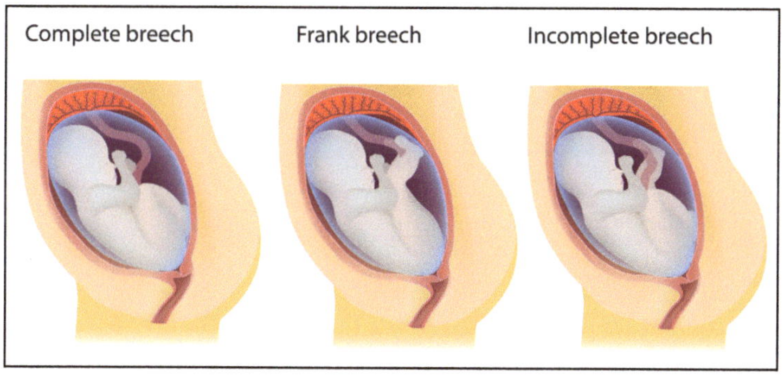

Shoulder Dystocia:

Causes: Small pelvis, big baby, female mutilation or tumor, narrow vaginal canal

Sx:

PE:

Dx: Turtle sign

______________________________ Tx:

____

____

Categories: 1. Problem of power - uterine contractions
2. Problem of passenger - macrosomia, position
3. Problem of passage - uterus or soft tissue abnormalities

Postpartum Hemorrhage: 4Ts: Tone, trauma, tissue (retained placental tissue), thrombin

Most common cause is UTERINE ATONY

- Uterine atony:
- Genital tract trauma:
- Retained placental tissue:
- Coagulation disorders:

Sx:

PE: Loss of > 500 mL within 24 hours after vaginal delivery
> 1000mL after C-section

Dx:

Tx:

Sheehan Syndrome:

Causes: Hemorrhage, hypotension, shock

Sx:

PE:

Dx:

Tx:

Cesarean Section: Surgical procedure to deliver baby/babies through the abdominal wall

Tx:

Endometritis: **Inflammation of endometrium (most common infection after childbirth)**

Risk Factors: C-section, PROM, vaginal delivery, D&C

Sx: Fever, tachycardia, foul smell

PE:

Dx:

Tx:

Perineal Lacerations: **Tearing of perineum during childbirth**

Sx:

PE: Depends on the degree of the tear/laceration

Dx:

Tx:

Puerperium or Postpartum Period: Lasts 6 weeks

- Placental implant site shrinks by ½ after delivery
- Lochia rubra: Normal postpartum discharge, blood, tissue, & decidua - stops after 5 or 6 weeks
- No vigorous exercise for 6-7 weeks
- Cervix shinks to 1 cm by the end of 1st week
- Vagina returns to antepartum condition by 3rd week
- Pelvic floor muscles return to original position, but are pre-disposed to cystocele, & rectocele
- Bladder capacity returns to normal by 6 weeks
- Ovulation can happen as early as 27 days after birth or 6 months if breastfeeding
    - Ovulation is suppressed by increased prolactin

Postpartum Depression:

Sx: Depressive symptoms that can start during pregnancy and last up to 12 months

PE:

Dx:

Tx:

Anorexia: *In Psych*

Vaginal Diseases/Infections: *In ID*

Premenstrual Dysphoric Disorder (PMDD): *In Psych*

Medications

______: MOA = ______
Indication(s)= ______
Side Effects = ______
Types/ Examples = ______

______: MOA = ______
Indication(s)= ______
Side Effects = ______
Types/ Examples = ______

______: MOA = ______
Indication(s)= ______
Side Effects = ______
Types/ Examples = ______

______: MOA = ______
Indication(s)= ______
Side Effects = ______
Types/ Examples = ______

______: MOA = ______
Indication(s)= ______
Side Effects = ______
Types/ Examples = ______

Medications

______________: MOA = ______________
Indication(s)= ______________
Side Effects = ______________
Types/ Examples = ______________

______________: MOA = ______________
Indication(s)= ______________
Side Effects = ______________
Types/ Examples = ______________

______________: MOA = ______________
Indication(s)= ______________
Side Effects = ______________
Types/ Examples = ______________

______________: MOA = ______________
Indication(s)= ______________
Side Effects = ______________
Types/ Examples = ______________

______________: MOA = ______________
Indication(s)= ______________
Side Effects = ______________
Types/ Examples = ______________

Neurology

Brain Anatomy
Worksheet

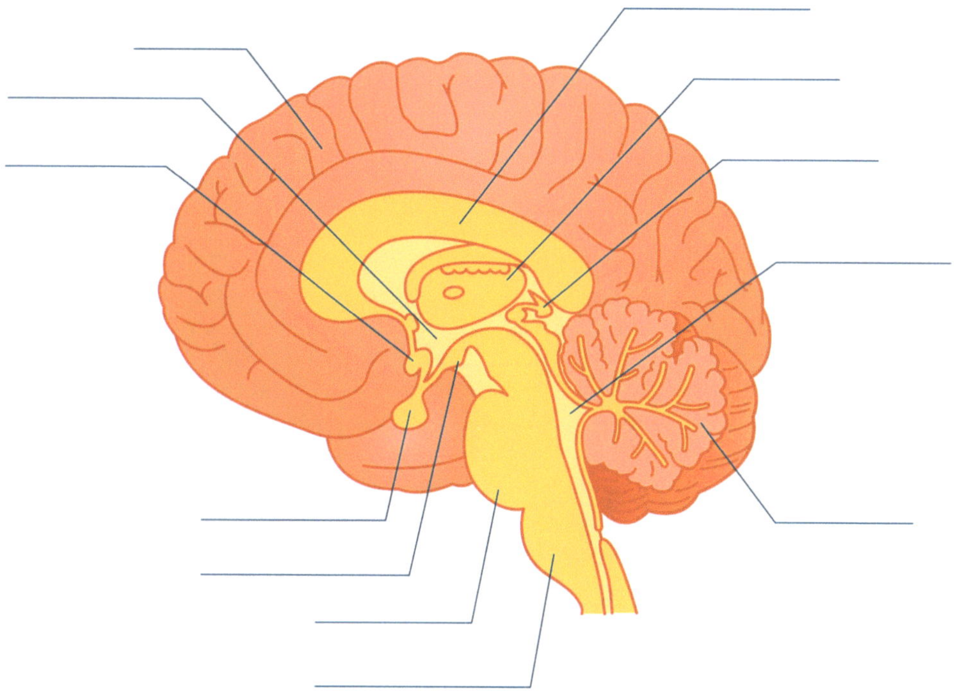

Mamillary body
Medulla Oblongata
Thalamus
Pineal Gland

Hypothalamus
Fourth Ventricle
Cerebellum
Cerebrum

Pituitary Gland
Corpus Callosum
Optic Chiasm
Pons

Peripheral Nerve Disorders

Complex Regional Pain Syndrome: **Chronic pain in a specific body region**

Most common = extremities

Sx: Pain, swelling, skin changes, vasomotor instability

PE:

Dx:

____

____

____

Tx:

Guillain-Barré Syndrome: **Associated with campylobacter jejuni**

Sx:

PE:

Dx: LP with increased CSF protein

Check vital capacity for lung function

____

____

____

Tx:

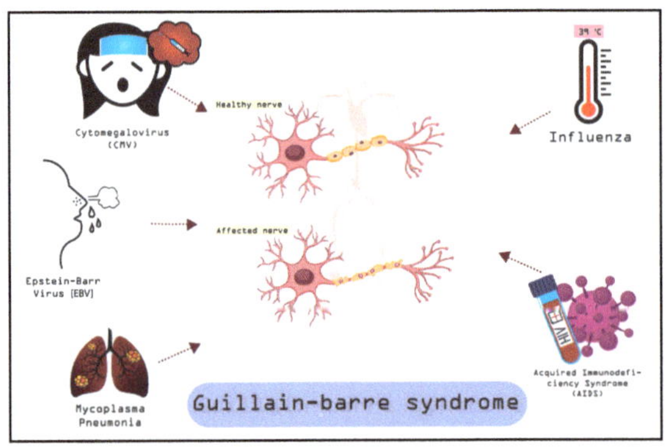

Peripheral Neuropathy:

Sx: Loss of sensation, paresthesia of extremities

PE:

Dx: EMG

____

____

____

Tx:

Diabetic Neuropathy: **Often associated with poor glycemic control**

Sx:

PE:

Dx: EMG

Tx:

Bell's Palsy: **CN VII - associated with HSV (prodrome viral illness)**

Sx:

PE: Paralysis of CN VII distribution, unable to lift eyebrow

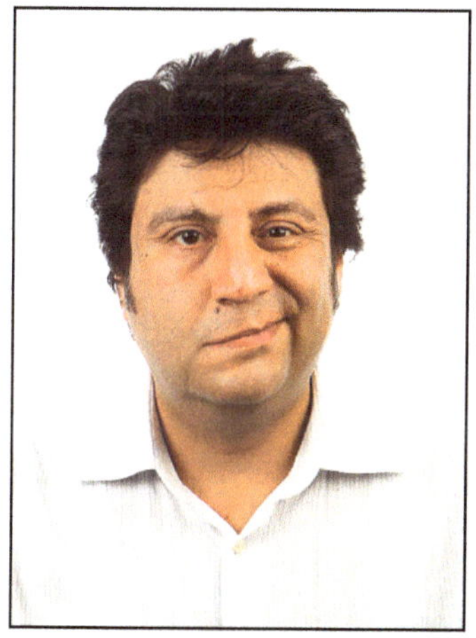

Dx:

Tx:

Trigeminal Neuralgia: **Demyelination & compression of CN V**

Sx: Intermittent zapping facial pain along CN V distribution

PE:

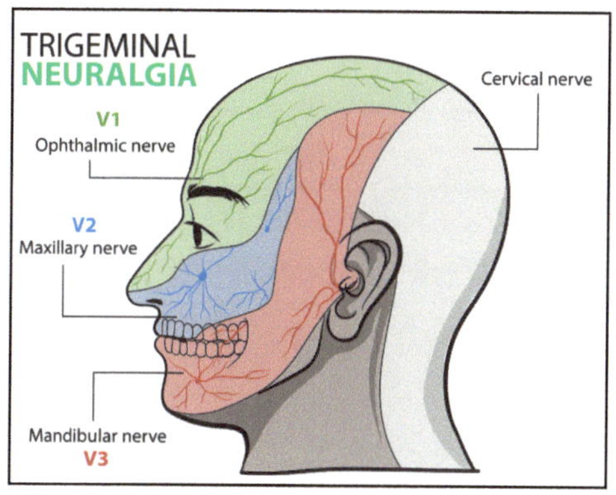

Dx:

Tx:

Movement Disorders

Essential Tremor: **Autosomal dominant - worse with caffeine, better with alcohol**

Sx:

PE:

Dx: Clinical

Tx:

Huntington's Disease: **Autosomal dominant**

Sx:

PE:

Dx: MRI = atrophy of basal ganglia

Tx:

Parkinson's Disease: **Low dopamine from substantia nigra**

Sx:

PE: Pill rolling, cogwheel rigidity, bradykinesia, shuffling gait, masked faces

Dx:

Tx:

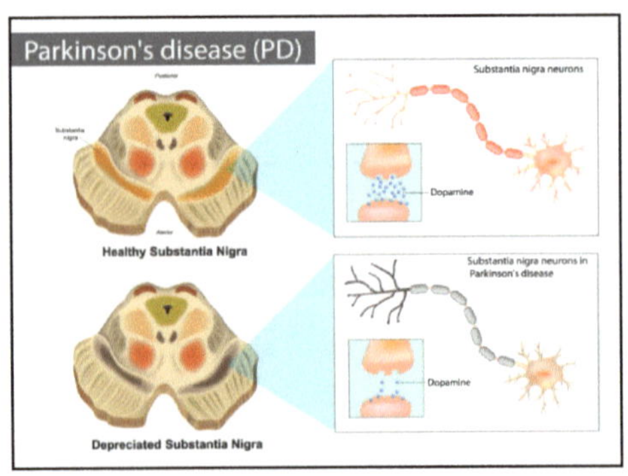

Infectious Neurologic Disorders

Encephalitis: **Viral infection of brain tissue**

Sx: Altered mental status, headache, seizures

PE:

Dx: Lumbar puncture

______________________________________ **Tx:**

____

____

Bacterial Meningitis:

Sx:

PE: + Kernig, + Brudzinski

Dx: LP = high protein, low glucose, high pressure

______________________________________ **Tx:**

____

____

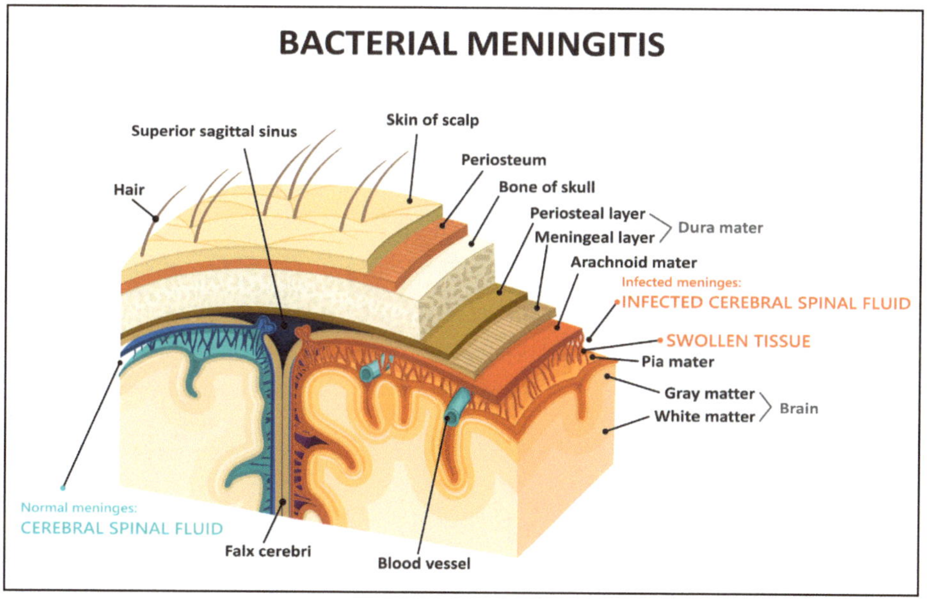

Viral Meningitis:

Sx:

PE:

Dx: LP + WBC, normal pressure & glucose

Tx:

Brain Abscess:

Sx: Headache, altered mental status, fever

PE:

Dx:

Tx:

Spine Disorders

Spinal Cord Compression: **Trauma**

Sx: Loss of motor/sensory reflexes depending on level of trauma to spinal cord

PE:

Dx:

Tx:

Brown-Séquard Syndrome: **Traumatic hemisection of spinal cord**

Sx: Ipsilateral loss vibration/proprioception - contralateral loss of pain/temp

PE:

Dx: MRI

Tx:

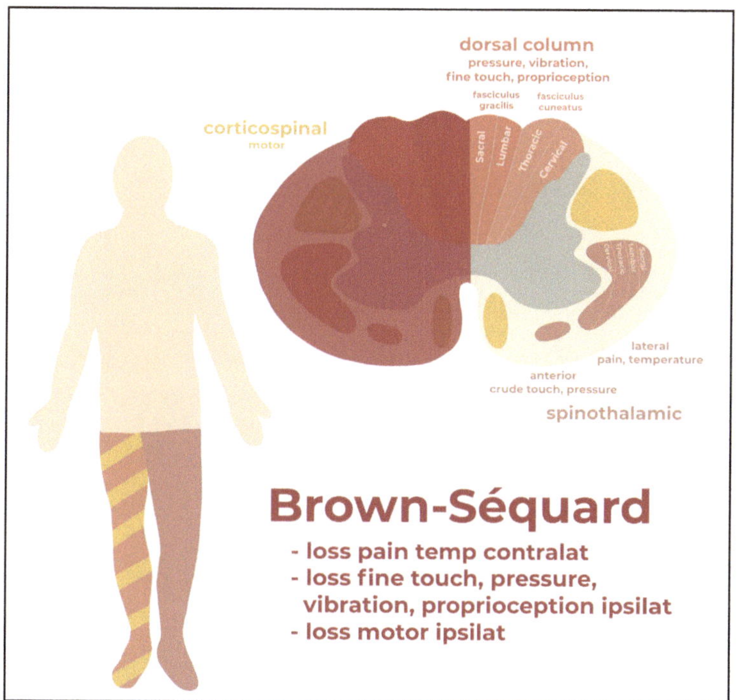

Neurocognitive & Neuromuscular Disorders

Delirium: Rapid onset, short-term, reversible

Sx: Acute, fluctuating change in mental status

PE:

Dx:

Tx:

Dementia: Gradual, irreversible memory loss

Alzheimer's: Most common cause

Sx:

Dx:

Tx:

Lewy Body: Parkinson's

Sx:

Dx:

Tx:

Frontotemporal: Personality/language changes (younger patients)

Sx:

Dx:

Tx:

Vascular: Correlated with cardiovascular disease

Sx:

Dx:

Tx:

Mild Cognitive Impairment: **No effect on ADLs**

Sx:

PE:

Dx: Montreal Cognitive Assessment (MoCa)

Tx:

Cerebral Palsy: **Trauma - hypoxia at birth**

Sx:

PE:

Dx: MRI of the brain

Tx:

Multiple Sclerosis: **Autoimmune**

Sx:

PE: Optic neuritis (Marcus-Gunn pupil)

Dx: LP = oligoclonal bands, MRI of spine

Tx:

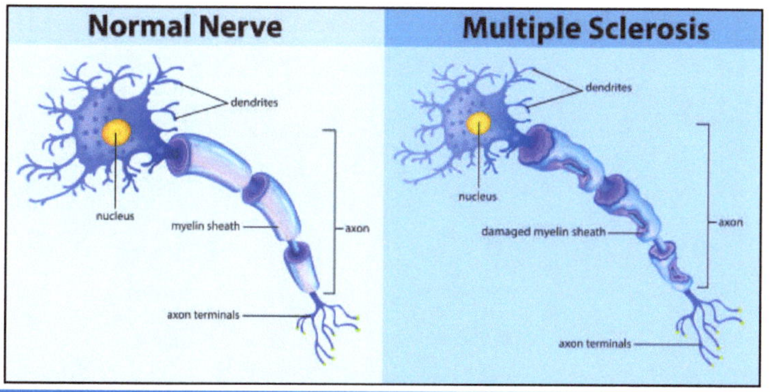

Myasthenia Gravis: Autoimmune

Sx: Muscles weaken and fatigue = hallmark of the disease: ptosis, diplopia

PE:

Dx: Ice bag test

Tx:

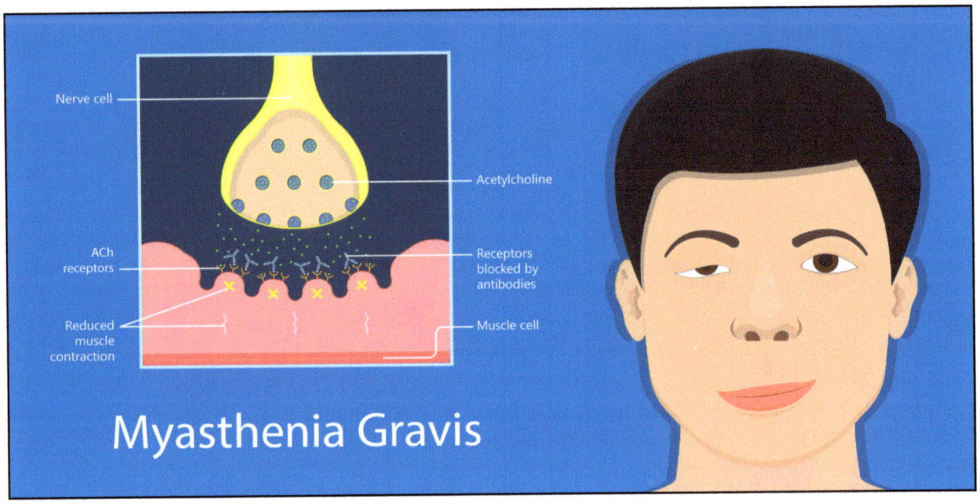

Emergent, Vascular, & Associated Neuro Disorders

Intracerebral Hemorrhage: Intraparenchymal bleeding

Sx:

PE:

Dx: Non-contrast head CT

Tx:

Epidural Hematoma: Arterial (middle meningeal artery)

Sx:

PE:

Dx: CT with biconvex lens

Tx:

Subdural Hematoma: Blood below dura (venous bridging veins)

Sx:

PE:

Dx: CT with crescent

Tx:

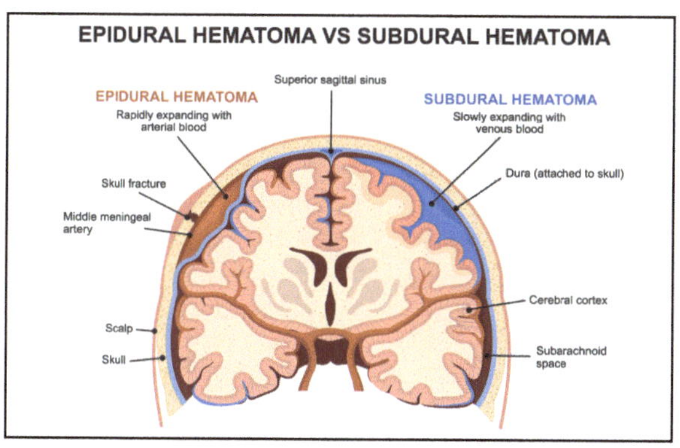

Subarachnoid Hemorrhage: **Ruptured aneurysm**

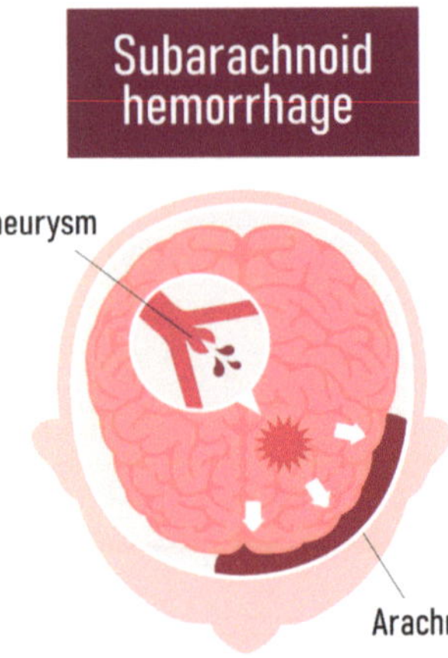

Sx: Thunderclap headache "worst headache of their life"

PE:

Dx: LP with xanthochromia

Tx:

Cerebral Aneurysm: **Weak, bulging spot of artery (AICA, PICA, MCA)**

Sx:

PE:

Dx: CTA

Tx:

Hydrocephalus: Accumulation of cerebral spinal fluid

Communicating:

Non-communicating:

Sx:

PE:

Dx: CT/MRI, US in infants

______________________________ **Tx:**

____

____

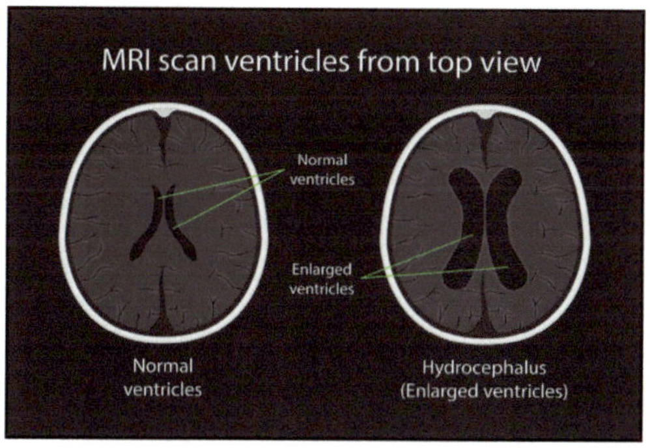

Normal Pressure Hydrocephalus: Enlarged ventricles with normal pressure

Sx: "Wacky, wobbly, wet"

PE:

Dx:

______________________________ **Tx:**

____

____

Idiopathic Intracranial Hypertension: High intracranial pressure

Sx:

PE:

Dx: LP with high opening pressure

______________________________ **Tx:**

____

____

Ischemic Stroke:

Sx:

PE:

Dx: Non-contrast head CT

Tx:

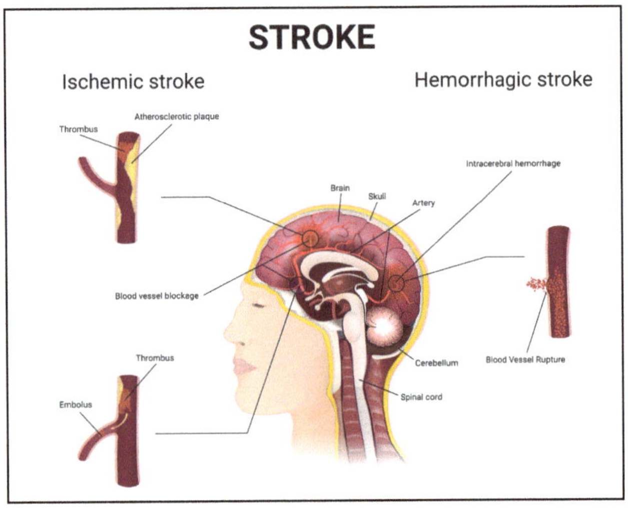

Vertebral **(vertigo)**

Basilar **(coma, CN palsy) – also affects PICA, AICA**

ACA **(leg weak, urinary incontinence)**

MCA **(face/arm weak, aphasia)**

PCA **(vision)**

Transient Ischemic Attack (TIA): Focal neural deficits that resolve within 1 hour

Sx:

PE:

Dx: Non-contrast head CT

Tx:

Syncope: **Loss of consciousness**

Sx:

PE:

Dx:

Tx:

Pituitary Apoplexy: **Infarct or hemorrhage of pituitary gland**

Sx:

PE:

Dx: CT/MRI

Tx:

Skull Fractures:

Sx:

PE: Battle sign, racoon eyes

Dx: CT

Tx:

Concussion:

Sx:

PE:

Dx: Glasgow Coma Scale

Tx:

Glasgow Coma Scale

Postconcussive Syndrome:

Sx: Headache, memory difficulties, fatigue

PE:

Dx:

Tx:

Traumatic Brain Injury (TBI):

Sx:

PE:

Dx: Serial Glasgow Coma Scale, non-contrast head CT

Tx:

Wernicke Encephalopathy: Thiamine deficiency associated with EtOH

Sx: Ataxia, confusion, nystagmus

PE:

Dx: MRI = punctate hemorrhages

Tx:

VP Shunt Malformation: Can lead to hydrocephalus

Sx:

PE:

Dx:

Tx:

Headaches

Cluster Headache: Unilateral

Sx: Ice pick headache lasting 15 minutes to 3 hours

PE:

Dx:

Tx:

Migraine Headaches: Unilateral

Sx: Throbbing pain, nausea, photophobia, +/- aura

PE:

Dx:

Tx:

Tension Headaches: Bilateral

Sx: Band-like pain around head

PE:

Dx:

Tx:

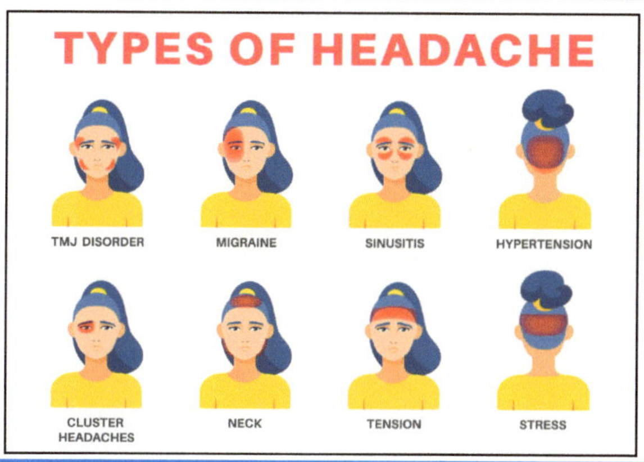

Congenital Neurologic Disorders

Chiari Malformation

Sx: Headache, imbalance, hydrocephalus

PE:

Dx: MRI

Seizure Disorders

Partial Seizure: Focal

Simple: No loss of consciousness

Complex: Loss of consciousness

Sx:

PE:

Dx: EEG

______________________________ **Tx:**

____

____

Generalized Seizures: Midbrain or brainstem

Tonic-colonic (grand mal) = rigid & convulsions

Sx:

PE:

Dx:

______________________________ **Tx:**

____

Absence (petite mal) = loss of consciousness without convulsions

Sx:

PE:

Dx:

______________________________ **Tx:**

____

Myoclonus = twitching, no loss of consciousness

Sx:

PE:

Dx:

______________________________ **Tx:**

____

Status Epilepticus: 5+ minutes of continuous seizures or 2+ separate seizures where there is not a recovery of consciousness

Sx:

PE:

Dx: Always check blood glucose

Tx:

Febrile Seizures: Convulsions with high temp > 38 °C

Sx:

PE:

Dx:

Tx:

Epilepsy: 2+ seizures, chronic, usually starts in childhood

Sx:

PE:

Dx:

Tx:

Misc. Neuro Concerns

Subclavian Steal Syndrome: Retrograde blood flow down ipsilateral vertebral artery

Sx: Hearing loss, tinnitus, changes in vision, vertigo, ataxia, syncope

PE:

Dx:

Tx:

Hemangioma: Benign vascular malformation

Sx:

PE:

Dx: Doppler US, MRI, or CT of hemangioma

Tx:

Glioblastoma: Aggressive form of brain cancer

Sx:

PE:

Dx: Brain MRI

Tx:

Giant Cell (Temporal) Arteritis: ***In Cardio***

Cauda Equina Syndrome: ***In MSK***

Spinal Epidural Abscess: ***In MSK***

Arteriovenous Malformation: ***In Cardiac***

Tourette Syndrome: ***In Psych***

Medications

______________: MOA = ______________
Indication(s)=______________
Side Effects = ______________
Types/ Examples = ______________

______________: MOA = ______________
Indication(s)=______________
Side Effects = ______________
Types/ Examples = ______________

______________: MOA = ______________
Indication(s)=______________
Side Effects = ______________
Types/ Examples = ______________

______________: MOA = ______________
Indication(s)=______________
Side Effects = ______________
Types/ Examples = ______________

______________: MOA = ______________
Indication(s)=______________
Side Effects = ______________
Types/ Examples = ______________

Medications

______________: MOA = ______________________________

Indication(s)=______________________________

Side Effects = ______________________________

Types/ Examples = ______________________________

____

____

______________: MOA = ______________________________

Indication(s)=______________________________

Side Effects = ______________________________

Types/ Examples = ______________________________

____

____

______________: MOA = ______________________________

Indication(s)=______________________________

Side Effects = ______________________________

Types/ Examples = ______________________________

____

____

______________: MOA = ______________________________

Indication(s)=______________________________

Side Effects = ______________________________

Types/ Examples = ______________________________

____

____

______________: MOA = ______________________________

Indication(s)=______________________________

Side Effects = ______________________________

Types/ Examples = ______________________________

____

____

Hematology

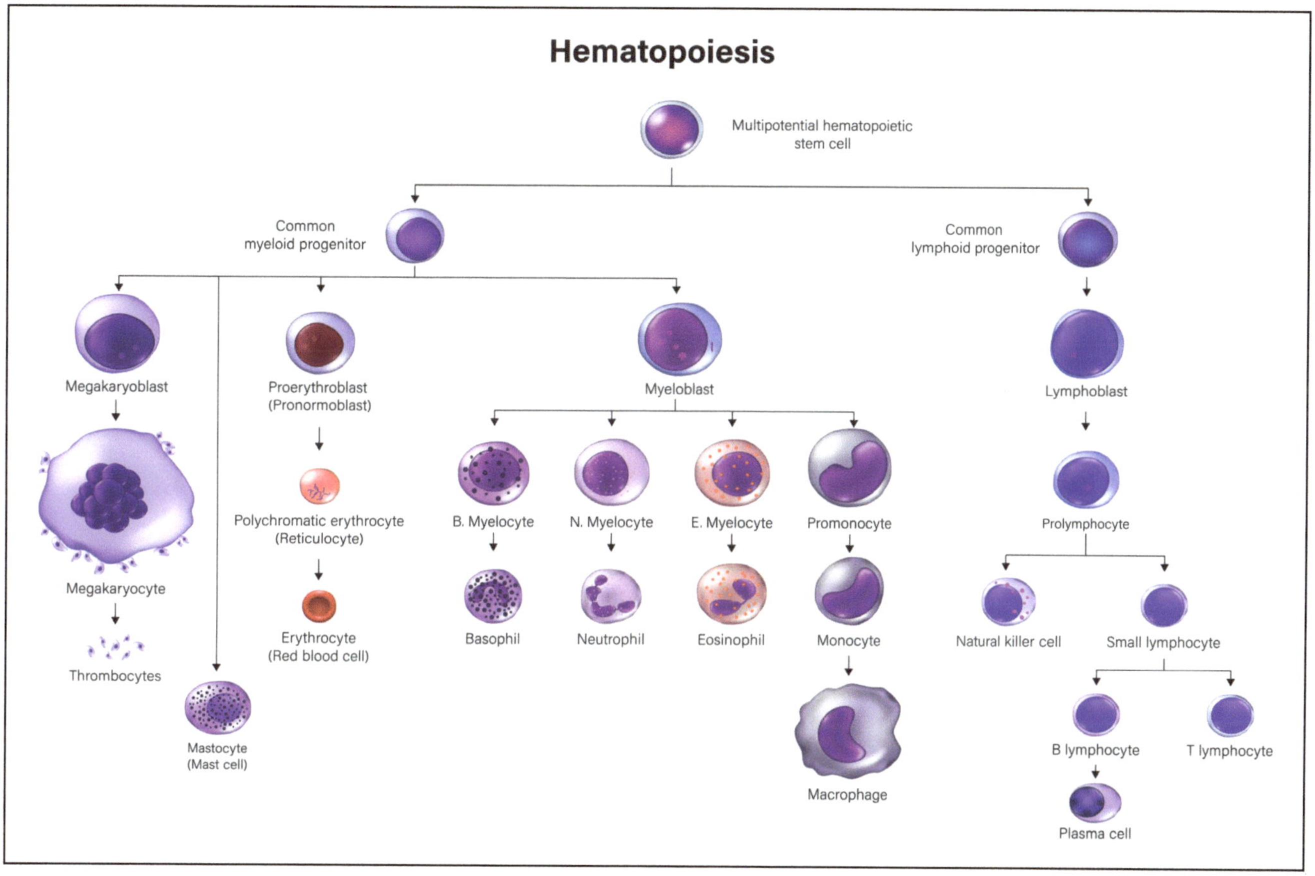
Hematopoiesis
Multipotential hematopoietic stem cell
Common myeloid progenitor
Common lymphoid progenitor
Megakaryoblast
Proerythroblast (Pronormoblast)
Myeloblast
Lymphoblast
Megakaryocyte
Polychromatic erythrocyte (Reticulocyte)
B. Myelocyte
N. Myelocyte
E. Myelocyte
Promonocyte
Prolymphocyte
Thrombocytes
Erythrocyte (Red blood cell)
Basophil
Neutrophil
Eosinophil
Monocyte
Natural killer cell
Small lymphocyte
Mastocyte (Mast cell)
Macrophage
B lymphocyte
T lymphocyte
Plasma cell

Anemias
Microcytic = low MCV < 80 fL

Iron Deficiency Anemia:

Sx:

PE: Fatigue, koilonychias, angular cheilitis

Dx:

Tx:

Thalassemia:

Alpha-Thalassemia: 4

Sx:

Dx: Hemoglobin, RBC, peripheral smear

Beta-Thalassemia: 2

Sx:

Dx: Same as above

Tx:

Alpha-Thalassemia	Beta-Thalassemia

Macrocytic: High MCV > 100 fL

Vitamin B12 Deficiency:

Causes: Veganism, pernicious anemia, bypass surgery

Sx: Glossitis, neuro symptoms

PE:

Dx: Labs = high MMA, high homocysteine

Tx:

Pernicious Anemia: **Can't absorb B12**

Sx:

PE:

Dx: + shilling test, CBC

Tx:

Folate Deficiency:

Causes: Alcoholism, pregnancy

Sx:

PE: Glossitis, neuro symptoms less common

Dx:

Tx:

Myelodysplastic Syndrome: **Precancerous - can lead to AML**

Sx:

PE: Labs = pancytopenia

Dx:

Tx:

Normocytic: Normal MCV 80 - 100 fL

Aplastic Anemia:

Sx:

PE: Petechiae, ecchymosis, weakness, pallor

Dx: Bone marrow biopsy

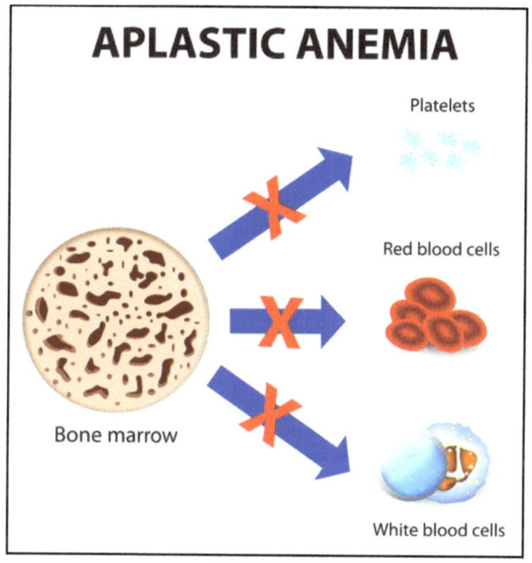

Tx:

Anemia of Chronic Disease: Micro - or normocytic anemia

Sx:

PE:

Dx: Low Fe, low TIBC, high ferritin

Tx:

Hemolytic Anemia:

Sx: Fatigue, jaundice

PE:

Dx: CBC, unconjugated (indirect) biliruben

Tx:

Autoimmune:

Causes: Idiopathic, CLL, autoimmune (SLE, RA, etc.)

Sx:

PE:

Dx: + Coombs

Tx:

Cold Ab Hemolytic Anemia:

Sx:

PE:

Dx: + Coombs

Tx:

Hereditary Spherocytosis: Red blood cells destroyed in spleen

Sx:

PE:

Dx: + Osmotic fragility, - Coombs

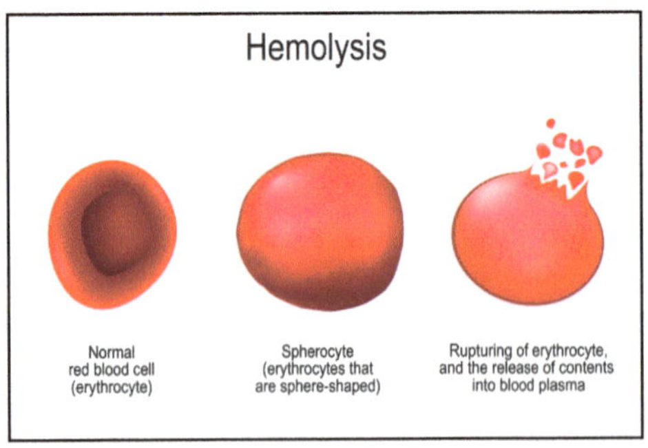

Tx:

Paroxysmal Nocturnal Hemoglobinuria (PNH): Idiopathic

Sx: Dark urine in the morning

PE:

Dx:

Tx:

G6PD Deficiency: X-linked recessive, patients with ancestry from Africa, Europe, and Asia

Sx:

PE:

Dx: + Heinz bodies & bite cells, - Coombs

Tx:

Sickle Cell Disease (Anemia): Autosomal recessive

Sx: Pain crisis, acute chest syndrome

PE:

Dx: Howell-Jolly bodies, high reticulocyte count

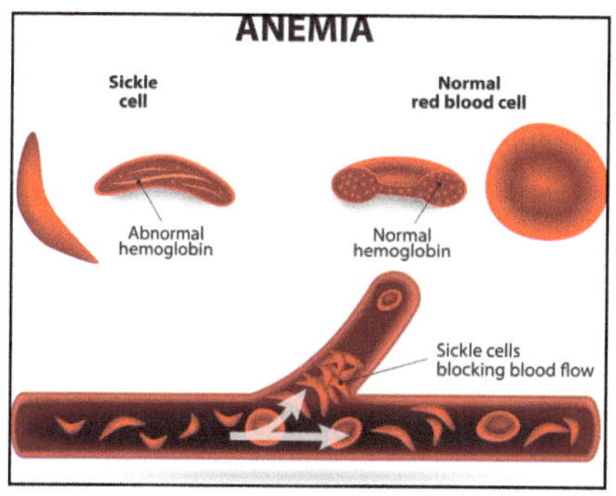

Tx:

Hematologic Malignancies

Hodgkin Lymphoma: **Bimodal age distribution, associated with EBV**

Sx:

PE:

Dx: Lymph node biopsy = Reed-Sternberg cells

____

____

____

Tx:

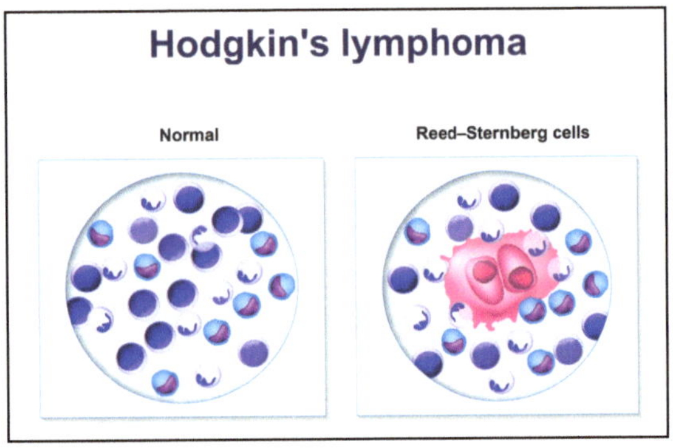

Non-Hodgkin Lymphoma: **Most common in patients > 50 years of age and with HIV, worse prognosis**

Sx:

PE:

Dx: Lymph node biopsy = Reed-Sternberg cells

____

____

____

Tx:

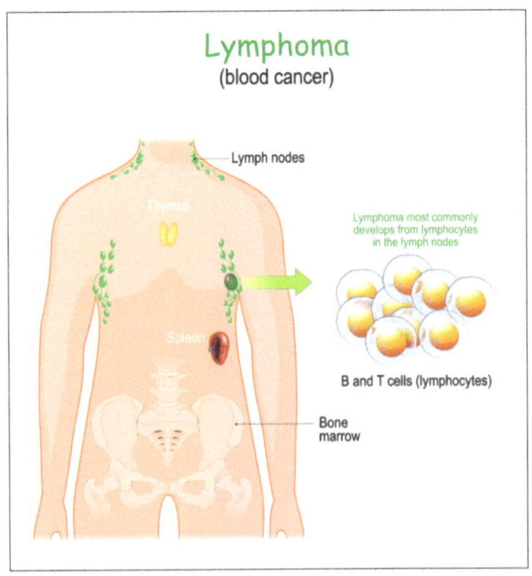

Acute Lymphocytic Leukemia (ALL): Seen in kids

Sx: Fever, bone pain, bruising, fatigue

PE:

Dx: CBC with differential, peripheral blood smear

Tx:

Acute Myeloid Leukemia (AML): Immature myeloid cell proliferation

Sx: Gingival hyperplasia

PE:

Dx: Bone marrow biopsy = Auer rods

Tx:

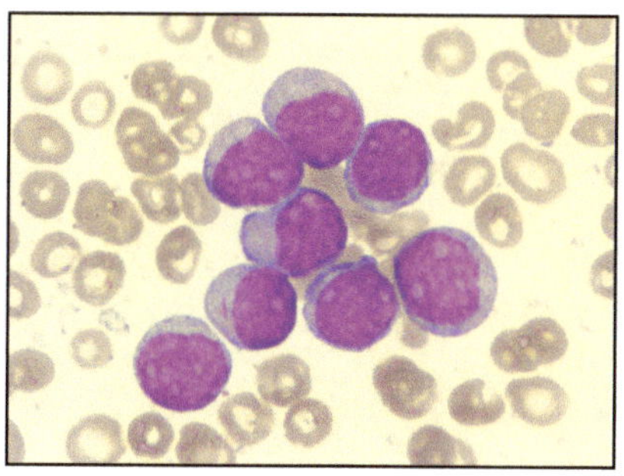

Chronic Lymphocytic Leukemia (CLL):

Sx:

PE:

Dx: High WBC, smudge cells

Tx:

Chronic Myeloid Leukemia (CML): Seen in adults

Sx:

PE:

Dx: Philadelphia chromosome

Tx:

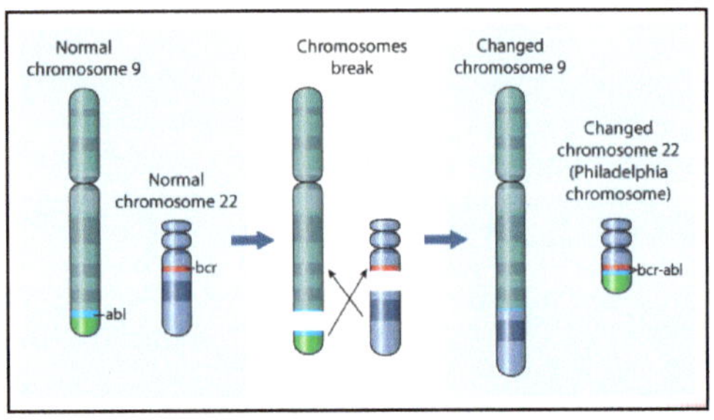

Multiple Myeloma (MM): Malignancy of plasma cells

Sx:

PE: UA - Bence Jones proteins
X-ray - lytic lesions

Dx:

Tx:

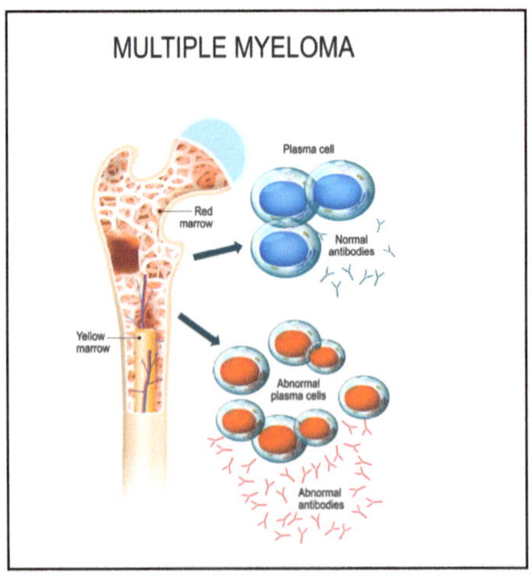

Clotting Pathway

von Willebrand Factor

Hypercoagulability Disorders

Protein C & S Deficiencies:

Complications: Pulmonary embolism & deep vein thrombosis

Sx:

PE:

Dx:

______________________________ **Tx:**

____

____

Factor V Leiden:

Complications: Pulmonary embolism & deep vein thrombosis

Sx:

PE:

Dx: CBC, other blood tests

______________________________ **Tx:**

____

____

Thrombocytopenias

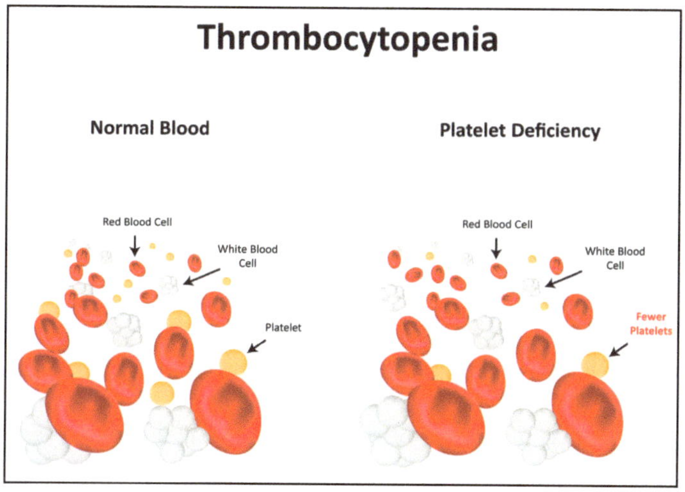

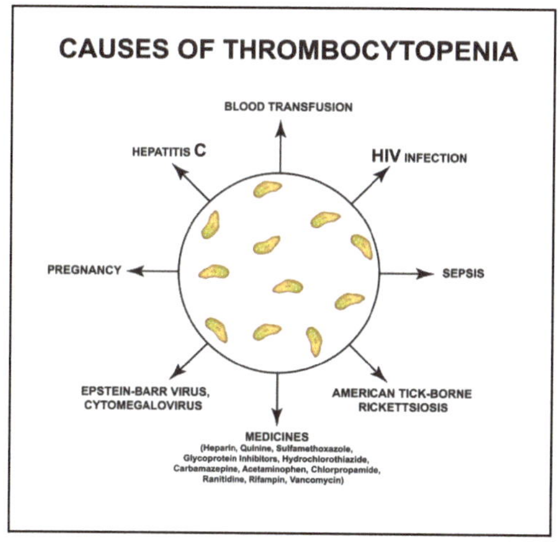

Idiopathic Thrombocytopenia Purpura (ITP): Autoimmune

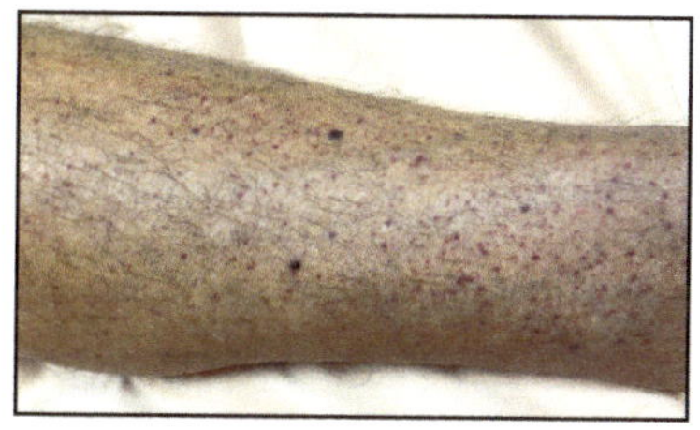

Sx:

PE:

Dx: Low platelets, normal PT & PTT, + Coombs

Tx:

Thrombotic Thrombocytopenia Purpura (TTP): ADAMTS13

Sx:

PE:

Dx: Pentad = thrombocytopenia, hemolytic anemia, renal failure, fever, neuro symptoms

Tx:

Hemolytic Uremic Syndrome (HUS): E. coli infection

Sx:

PE:

Dx: Triad = thrombocytopenia, hemolytic anemia, renal failure

Tx:

Disseminated Intravascular Coagulation (DIC): Simultaneous clot formation & breakdown

Sx: Thrombosis, excessive bleeding

PE:

Dx:

Tx:

Heparin-Induced Thrombocytopenia (HIT):

Sx:

PE:

Dx: Increased bleeding time, normal PT & PTT

Tx:

Bleeding Disorders

Hemophilia A (VIII) & B (IV-Christmas): **X-linked recessive**

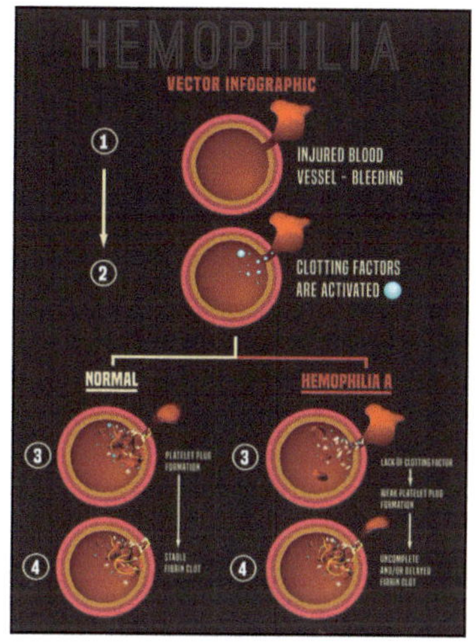

Sx:

PE:

Dx: Factor assay, long PTT

Tx:

Hemophilia C (XI): **Autosomal recessive - more common in patients of Ashkenazi Jewish ancestry**

Sx:

PE:

Dx: Prolonged PTT

Tx:

Von Willebrand Disease (vWB): **Autosomal dominant - more common in women**

Sx:

PE:

Dx: Low vWB, long bleeding time, long PTT

Tx:

Myeloproliferative Disorders

Primary Polycythemia Vera: **Marrow malignancy with RBC overproduction**

Sx: Pruritis after shower

PE:

Dx: JAK2 mutation, high hemoglobin & hematocrit

Tx:

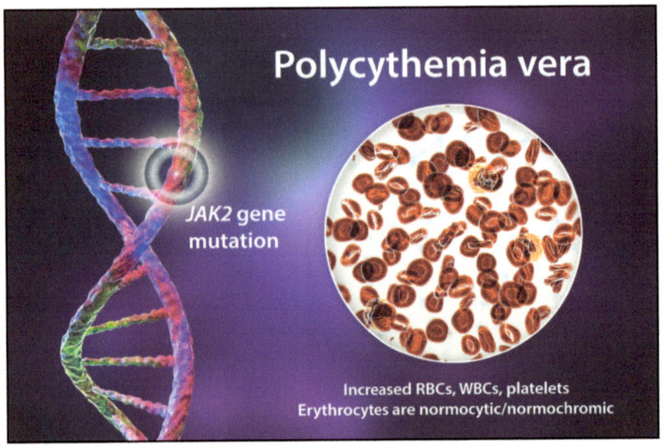

Thrombocythemia: **Overproduction of platelets**

Sx: Headache, nausea, vomiting, dizziness, thrombosis

PE:

Dx:

Tx:

Hemochromatosis: Autosomal recessive

Complications: Cirrhosis, liver cancer, diabetes mellitus, CHF, arthritis

Sx:

PE:

Dx: Labs:

Liver biopsy:

Tx:

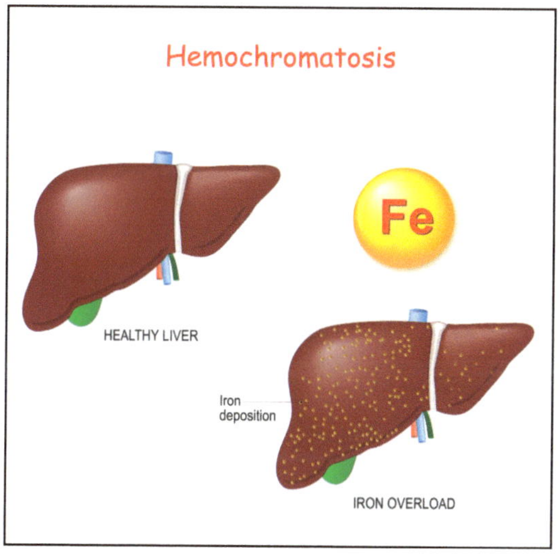

Hemostatis:

Definition:

Explanation:

Medications

______________: MOA = ______________________________
Indication(s)=______________________________
Side Effects = ______________________________
Types/ Examples = ______________________________
____
____

______________: MOA = ______________________________
Indication(s)=______________________________
Side Effects = ______________________________
Types/ Examples = ______________________________
____
____

______________: MOA = ______________________________
Indication(s)=______________________________
Side Effects = ______________________________
Types/ Examples = ______________________________
____
____

______________: MOA = ______________________________
Indication(s)=______________________________
Side Effects = ______________________________
Types/ Examples = ______________________________
____
____

______________: MOA = ______________________________
Indication(s)=______________________________
Side Effects = ______________________________
Types/ Examples = ______________________________
____
____

Medications

____________________: MOA = ____

Indication(s)=____

Side Effects = ____

Types/ Examples = ____

____________________: MOA = ____

Indication(s)=____

Side Effects = ____

Types/ Examples = ____

____________________: MOA = ____

Indication(s)=____

Side Effects = ____

Types/ Examples = ____

____________________: MOA = ____

Indication(s)=____

Side Effects = ____

Types/ Examples = ____

____________________: MOA = ____

Indication(s)=____

Side Effects = ____

Types/ Examples = ____

Renal, GU, Electrolytes

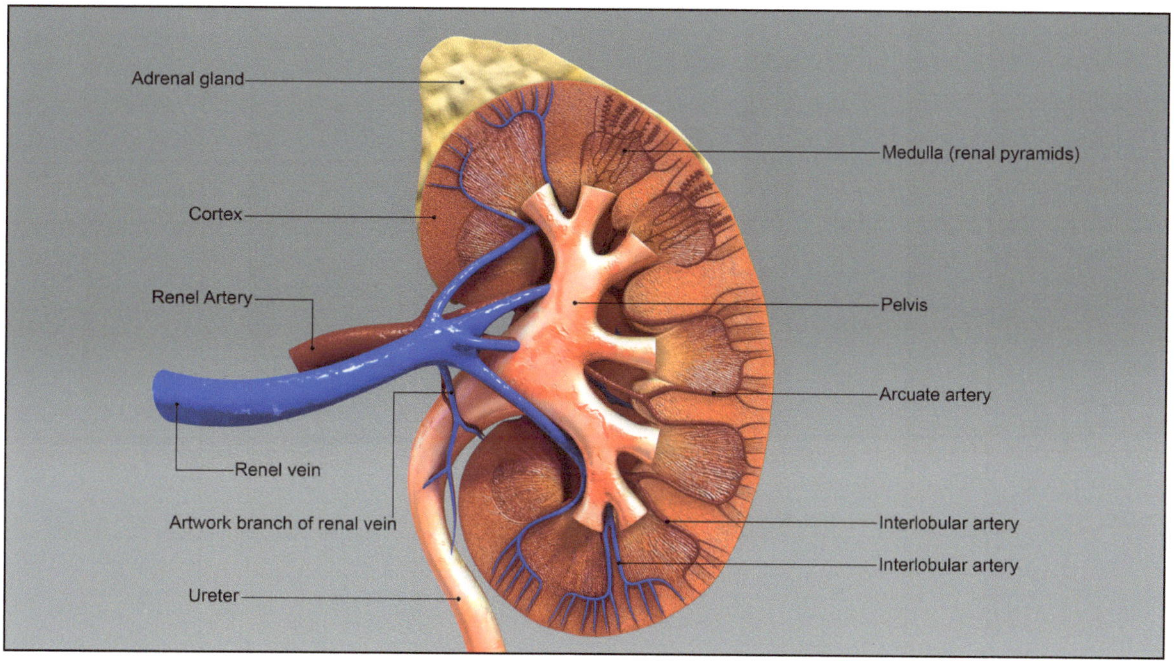

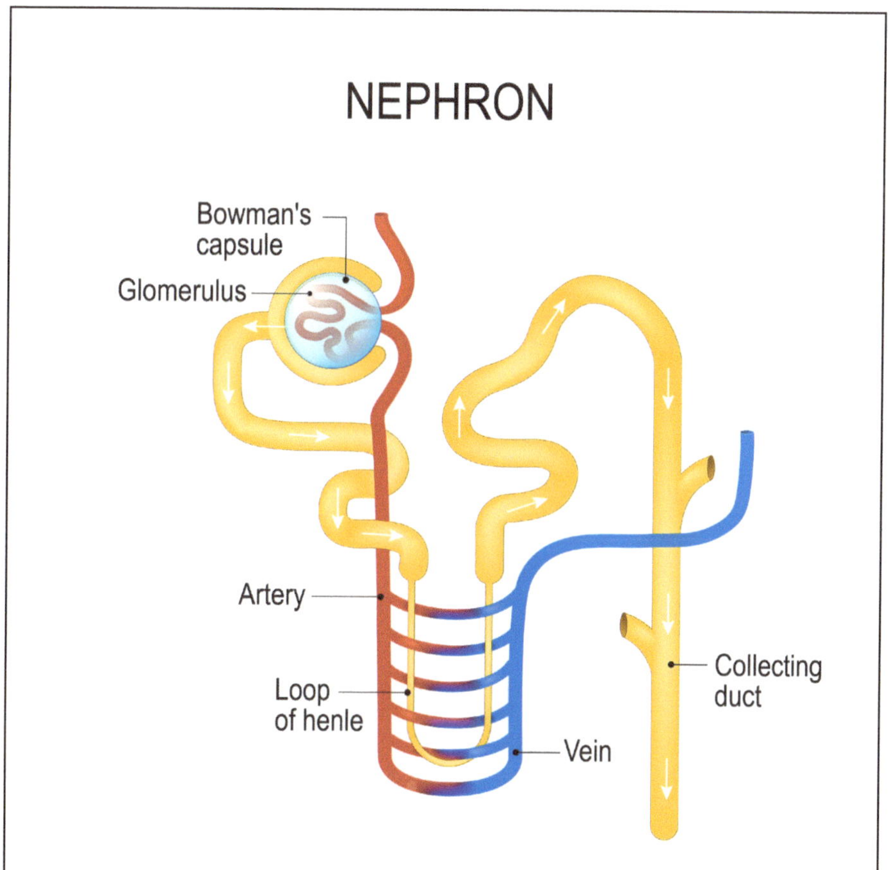

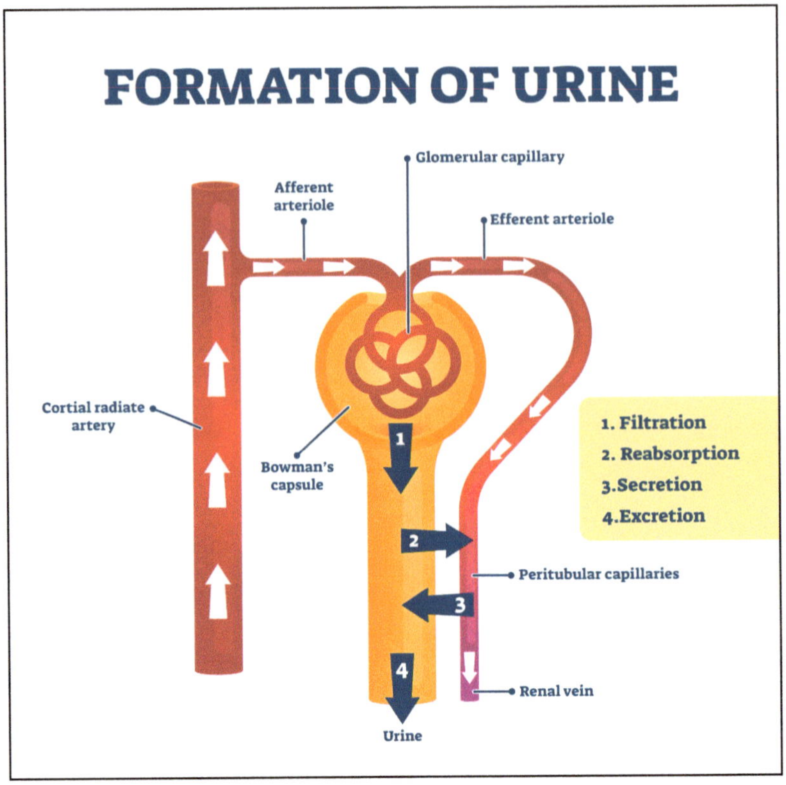
FORMATION OF URINE
Glomerular capillary
Afferent arteriole
Efferent arteriole
Cortial radiate artery
Bowman's capsule
1. Filtration
2. Reabsorption
3.Secretion
4.Excretion
Peritubular capillaries
Renal vein
Urine
1
2
3
4

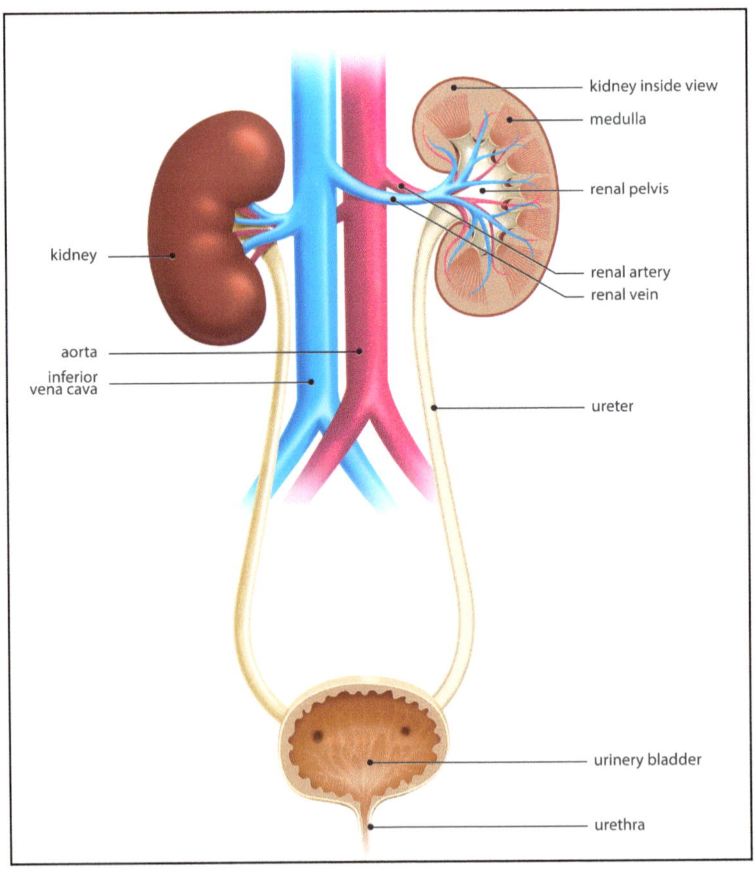
kidney inside view
medulla
renal pelvis
kidney
renal artery
renal vein
aorta
inferior vena cava
ureter
urinery bladder
urethra

Acute Kidney Injury

Pre-Renal: **Decreased perfusion (hypovolemia), renal artery stenosis**

Sx:

PE:

Dx: BUN:Cr > 20:1, high osmolality, low FENa

Tx:

Post-Renal: **Obstruction, BPH, tumor, stone**

Sx:

PE:

Dx:

Tx:

Intra-Renal: **Damage to kidney parenchyma**

Sx:

PE:

Dx: BUN:Cr < 15:1, low osmolality, high FENa

Tx:

Acute Tubular Necrosis: Ischemia, drugs, rhabdomyolysis

Sx:

PE:

Dx: Muddy brown casts

Tx:

Acute Interstitial Nephritis: Infection (strep), drugs (NSAIDs), autoimmune (SLE)

Sx: Arthralgia, fever, rash, WBC casts, eosinophilia

PE:

Dx:

Tx:

Nephrotic Syndrome

Proteinuria > 3.5 g/24-hr, edema, hypoalbuminemia, hyperlipidemia, oval fat bodies

---

Minimal Change Disease: **Idiopathic - usually seen in kids**

Sx:

PE:

Dx: Children = clinical, adults = biopsy

Tx:

Membranous Nephropathy:

Sx:

PE:

Dx: Biopsy

Tx:

Focal Segmental Glomerulosclerosis: **Most common in black patients**

Sx: Primary (idiopathic)
Secondary (HIV, heroin, obesity)

PE:

Dx:

Tx:

Nephritic Syndrome

Glomerulus inflammation - hematuria, oliguria, hypertension from sodium retention

Damage to the basement membrane

Acute Glomerulonephritis:

Sx: Hematuria, proteinuria, decreased GFR, increased blood pressure, edema

PE:

Dx:

____

____

____

Tx:

Post-Strep Glomerulonephritis: Post strep infection

Sx: Periorbital edema

PE:

Dx:

____

____

____

Tx:

IgA Nephropathy (Berger): Most common in East Asian patients

Sx:

PE:

Dx:

Tx:

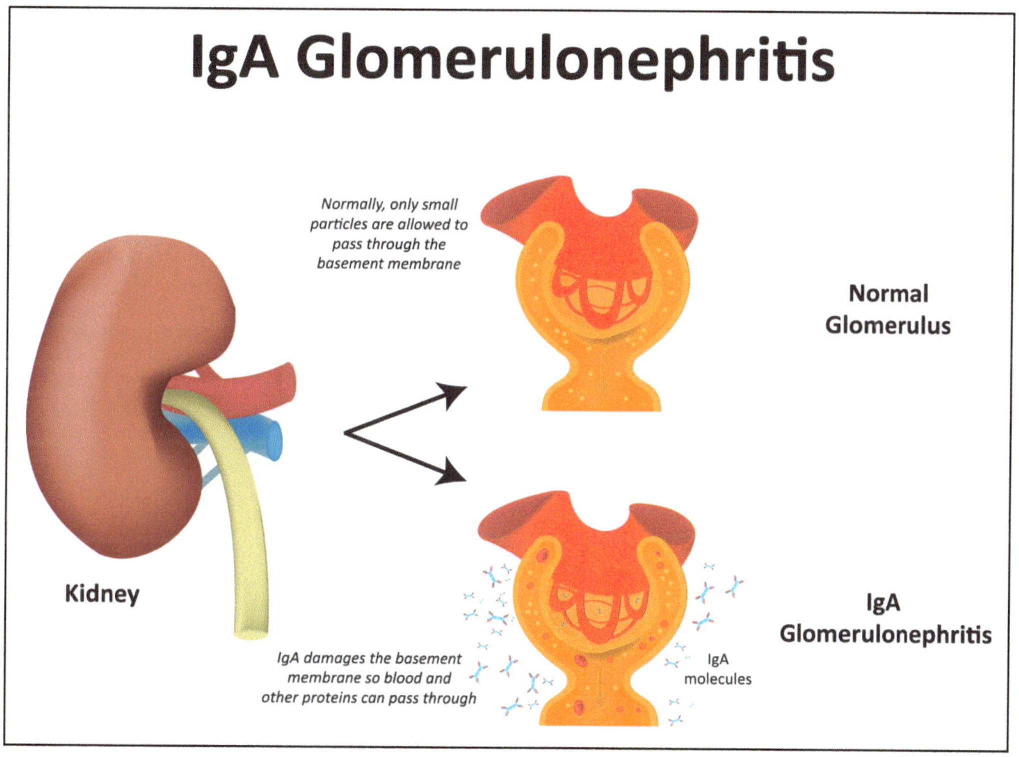

Membranous Glomerulonephritis (MGN): Mostly idiopathic

Sx:

PE:

Dx:

Tx:

Goodpasture Syndrome:

Sx: Hemoptysis

PE:

Dx: Biopsy linear deposits (anti-GBM)

Tx:

Chronic Kidney Disease: Low GFR > 3 months

Causes: Diabetes, hypertension

Sx: MAD HUNGER

PE:

Dx:

Tx:

M

A

D

H

U

N

G

E

R

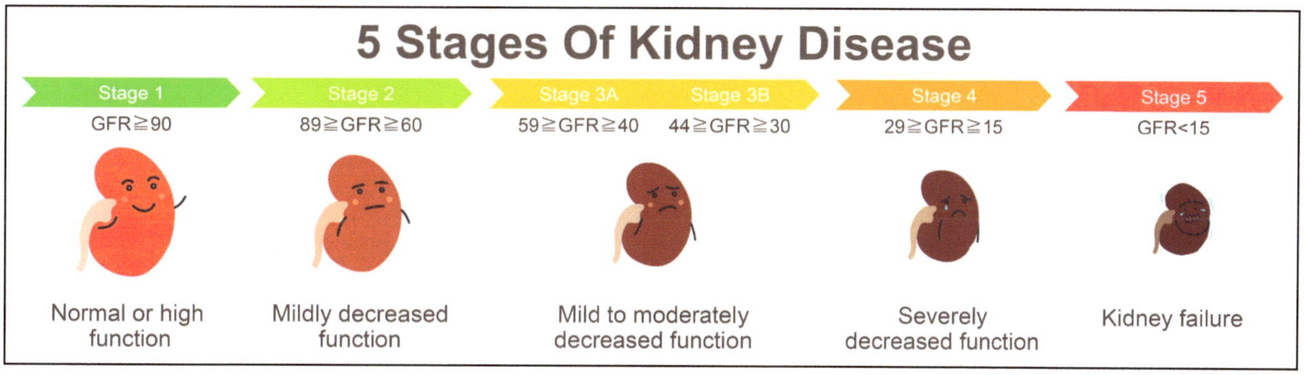

Acid Base Disorders

Metabolic Acidosis: **Anion gap = Na- (CL + HC03) < 11**

Anion gap - Sx:

PE:

Dx:

M
U
D
P
I
L
E
S

Non-Anion gap - Sx:

PE:

Dx:

Tx:

Metabolic Alkalosis:

Causes: Vomiting, diuretics, Cushing's

Sx:

PE:

Dx:

Tx:

Respiratory Acidosis:

Causes: Hypoventilation, COPD, opiates

Sx:

PE:

Dx:

Tx:

Respiratory Alkalosis:

Causes: Hyperventilation, pregnancy, anxiety

Sx:

PE:

Dx:

Tx:

Electrolyte Imbalance

Hyponatremia: < 135 mEq/L

Sx: Acute = headache, N/V

Chronic = ataxia

PE:

Dx:

Tx:

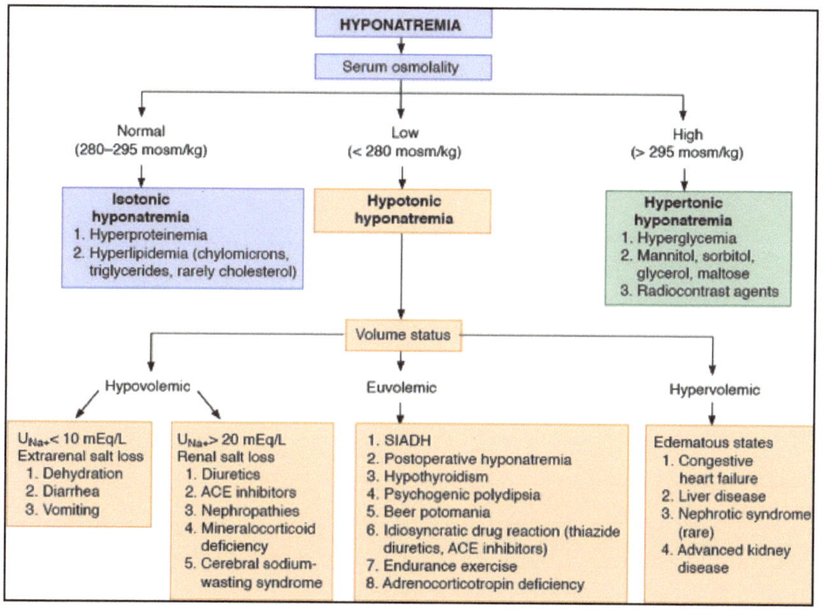

Hypernatremia: > 145 mEq/L

Causes: Dehydration, diabetes insipidus

Sx:

PE:

Dx:

Tx:

Hypokalemia: < 3.5 mmol/L

Causes: Diuretics, hyperaldosteronism

Sx:

PE: EKG = flat T waves, U waves, Torsades

Dx:

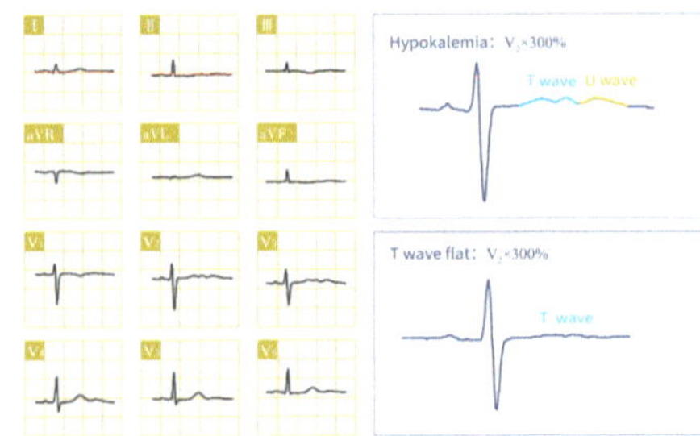

Hypokalemia

T wave is flat. T wave amplitude=U wave amplitude

Tx:

Hyperkalemia: > 5 mmol/L

Causes: DKA, renal failure, ACE/ARB

Sx:

PE: EKG = peaked T waves, sine wave

Dx:

Tx:

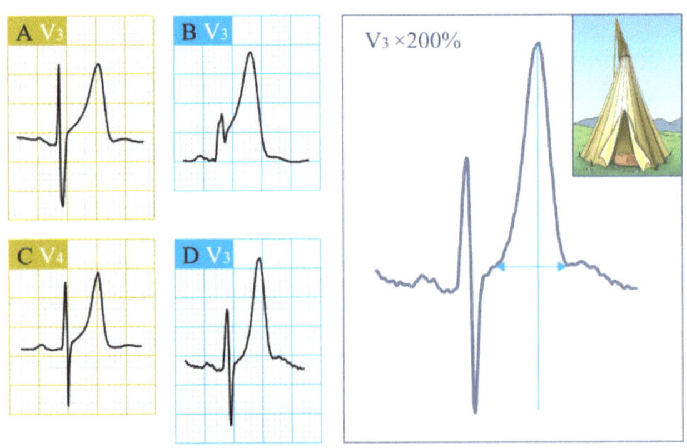

High T wave

Illustration A and Illustration C are normal high amplitude T waves.
Illustration B is a hyperacute T wave.
Illustration D is the T wave of hyperkalemia.

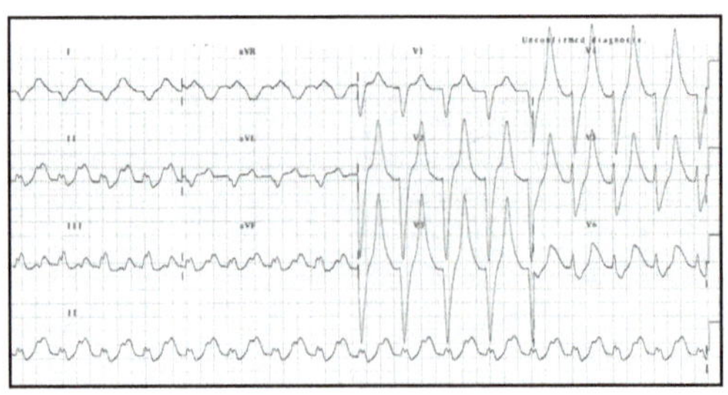

Hypocalcemia: < 8.5 mg/dL total

Causes: CKD, hypoparathyroidism, pancreatitis

Sx:

PE: EKG = long QT

Dx:

Tx:

Hypercalcemia: > 10.5 mg/dL total

Causes: Hyperparathyroidism, malignancy, thiazides

Sx:

PE: EKG = short QT

Dx:

Tx:

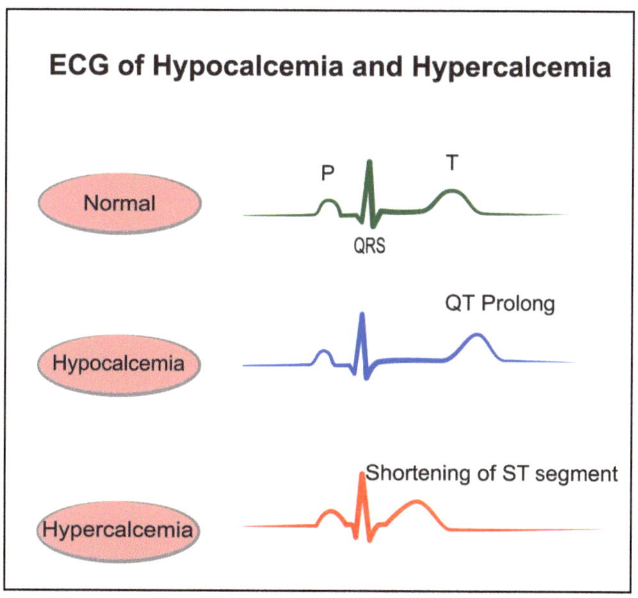

Hypomagnesemia: < 1.8 mg/dL

Causes: Diuretics, alcohol, PPI

Sx:

PE: Long QT, torsades

Dx:

Tx:

Hypermagnesemia:

Cause: CKD

Sx:

PE: EKG = peaked T waves

Dx:

Tx:

Hypovolemia	Isovolumia	Hypervolemia

Renal & GU Infections

Cystitis: Bladder infection (most common cause is E. coli)

Sx:

PE:

Dx: UA

____

____

____

Tx:

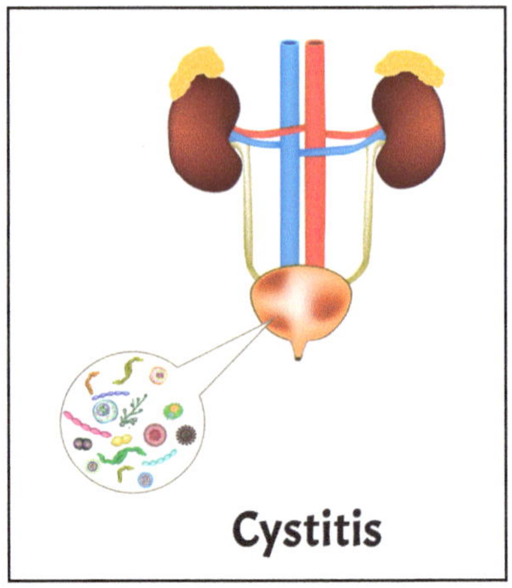

Epididymitis: Chlamydia/gonorrhea < 35 years old, E. coli > 35 years old

Sx:

PE: + Cremasteric reflex, + Prehn's

Dx:

____

____

____

Tx:

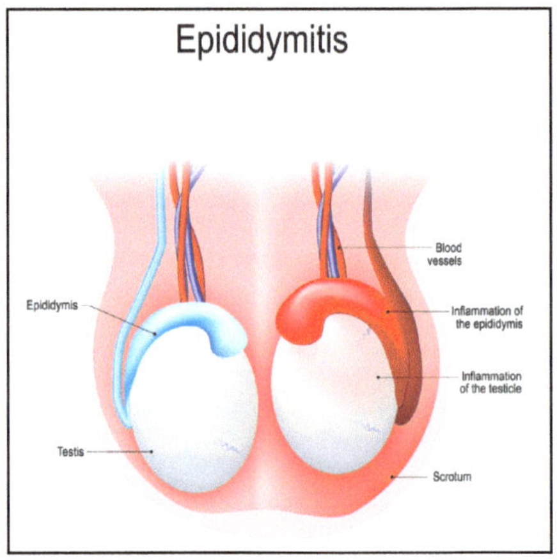

Orchitis: Most common cause is mumps

Sx:

PE:

Dx:

____

____

____

Tx:

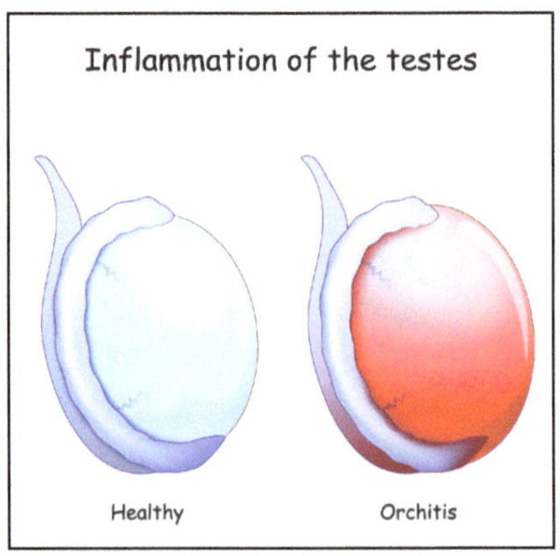

Prostatitis: Chlamydia/gonorrhea < 35 years old, E. coli > 35 years old

Sx:

PE:

Dx: Digital rectal exam

Tx:

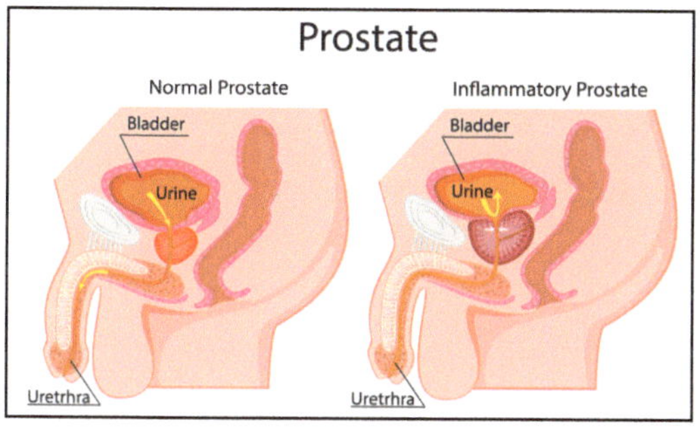

Pyelonephritis: UTI that ascends ureters to kidneys

Sx:

PE: Flank pain and/or CVA tenderness

Dx:

Tx:

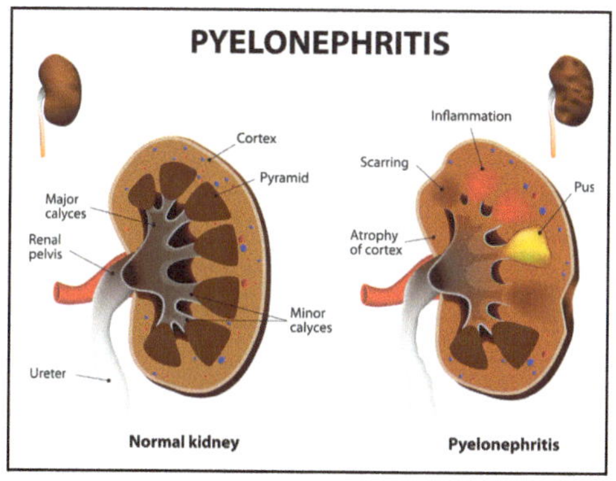

Urethritis: Most common STI

Sx: Dysuria, discharge

PE:

Dx:

Tx:

Other Kidney Disorders

Nephrolithiasis: **Most common calcium oxalate**

Sx:

PE:

Dx: CT (without contrast)
US if pregnant

Tx:

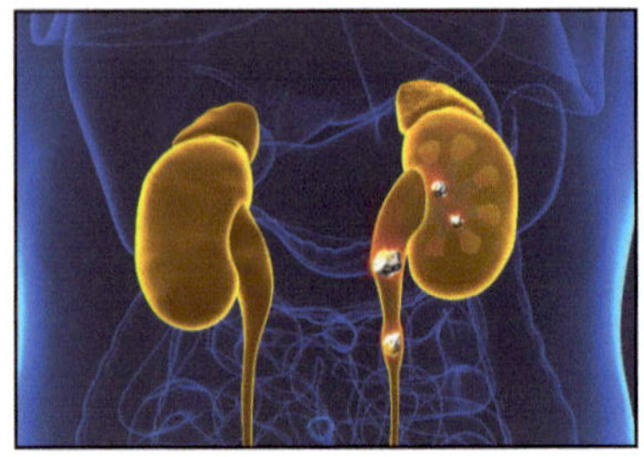

Hydronephrosis: **Dilation of renal pelvis**

Sx:

PE:

Dx: US then CT

Tx:

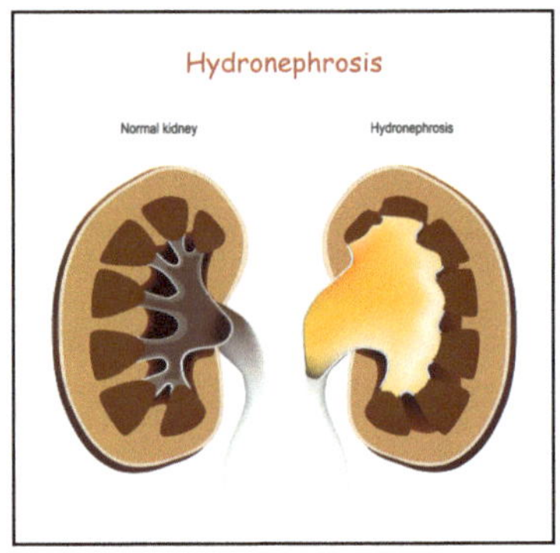

Polycystic Kidney Disease: **Autosomal dominant**

Sx: Many people are asymptomatic, HTN, hematuria

PE:

Dx:

Tx:

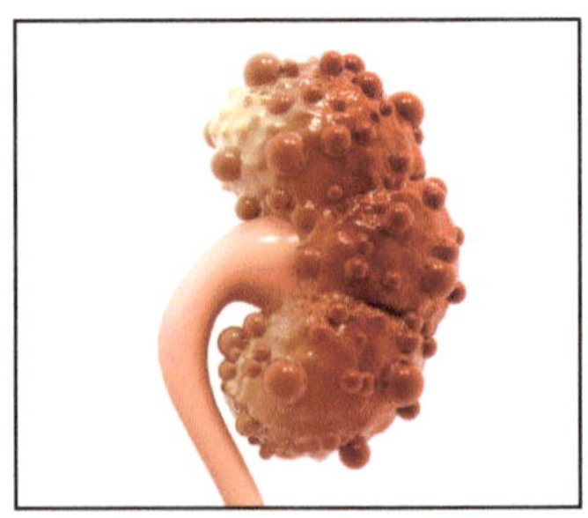

Renal Arterial Stenosis: Narrow renal artery

Sx:

PE: Bruit

Dx: Renal arteriography

Tx:

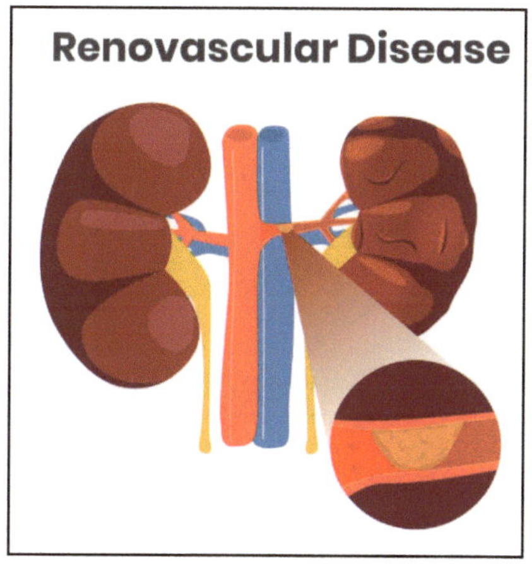

Vesicoureteral Reflux: Increased risk for UTI & pyelonephritis

Sx:

PE:

Dx: Renal US, voiding cystourethrogram (VCUG)

Tx:

Horseshoe Kidney: Most common renal fusion anomaly

Sx:

PE:

Dx: US (usually antenatal)

Tx:

Kidney & GU Carcinomas

Wilms' Tumor: **Nephroblastoma in children**

Sx: Abdominal mass/swelling

PE:

Dx:

Tx:

Bladder Cancer: **Most common cause = smoking**

Sx:

PE:

Dx: Cystoscopy

Tx:

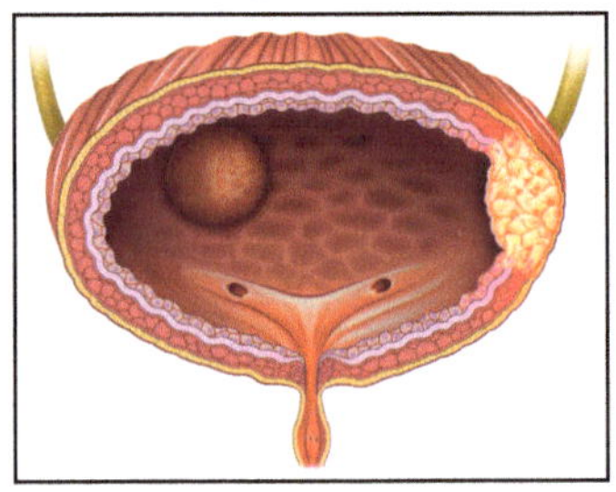

Prostate Cancer: **Most common adenocarcinoma**

Sx:

PE:

Dx: Biopsy, MRI, high PSA

Tx:

Screening:

Renal Cell Carcinoma:

Sx: Flank pain, hematuria, mass

PE:

Dx:

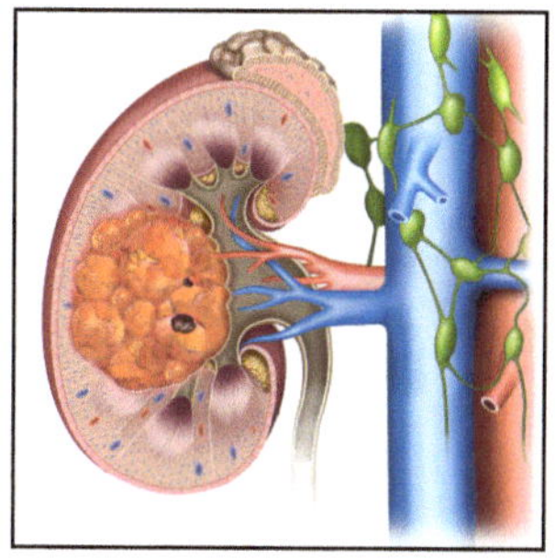

Tx:

Testicular Cancer:

Risk Factor: Cryptorchidism

Sx:

PE:

Dx: US, monitor with alpha-fetoprotein

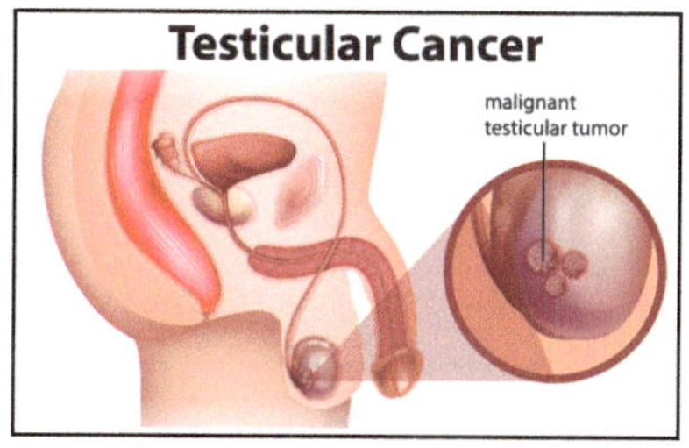

Tx:

Penile Cancer:

Sx: Painless lump or ulcer, lymphadenopathy

PE:

Dx: Biopsy

Tx:

Incontinence Disorders

Stress Incontinence: Coughing, laughing, jumping

Sx:

Dx:

Tx:

Urge Incontinence: Overactive detrusor muscle

Sx:

Dx:

Tx:

Overflow Incontinence: Neurological condition, blockage, or elderly

Sx:

Dx:

Tx:

Mixed Incontinence: Stress + Urge

Sx:

Dx:

Tx:

Functional Incontinence: Physical or mental disabilities

Sx:

Dx:

Tx:

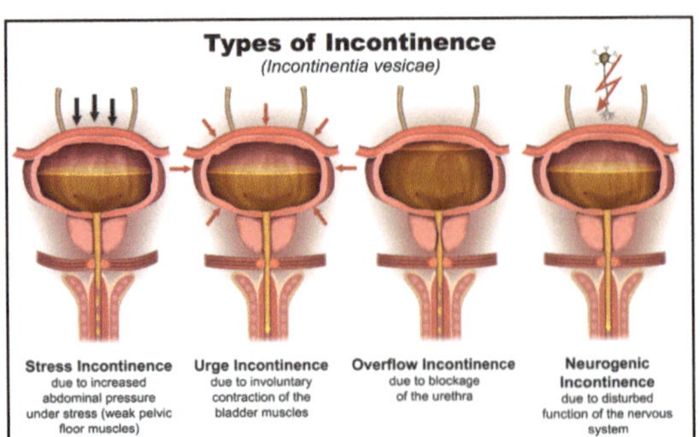

Male Genitalia Concerns

Hydrocele:

Sx:

PE:

Dx: Scrotal US

Tx:

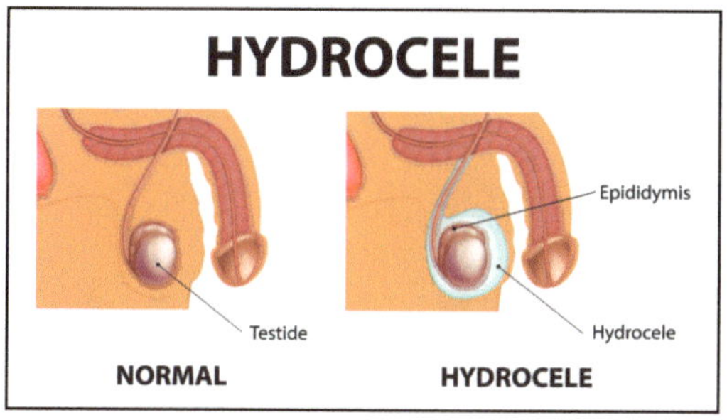

Spermatocele: **Epididymal cyst filled with sperm**

Sx:

PE:

Dx:

Tx:

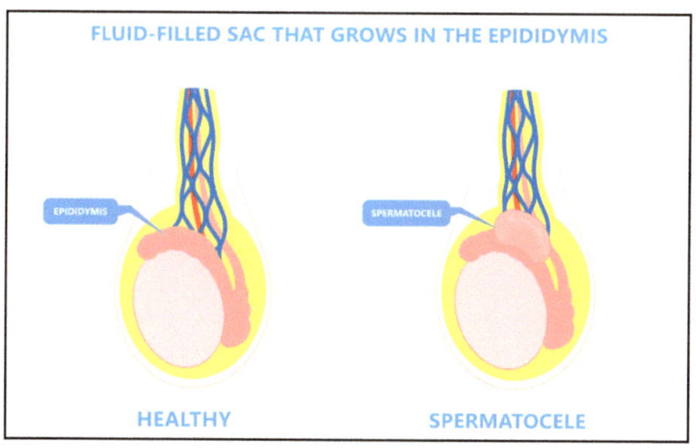

Varicocele: Dilation of pampiniform plexus

Sx:

PE: "Bag of worms"

Dx:

Tx:

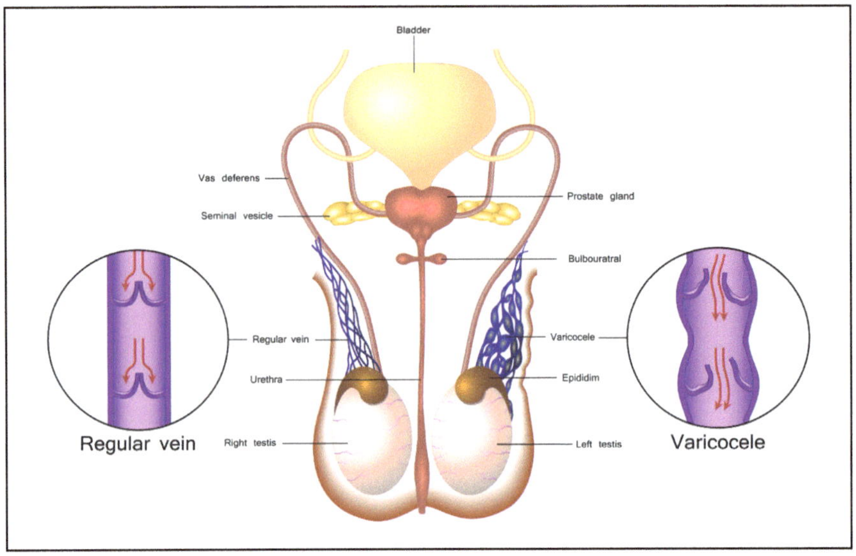

Testicular Torsion: **Acute twisting of spermatic cord EMERGENCY!**

Sx:

PE: Cremasteric reflex absent, bell clapper deformity (predisposition)

Dx:

Tx:

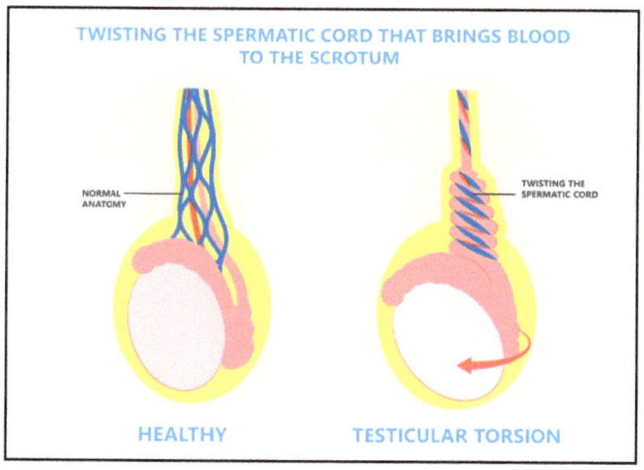

Cryptorchidism: **Undescended testicles**

Sx:

PE:

Dx:

Tx:

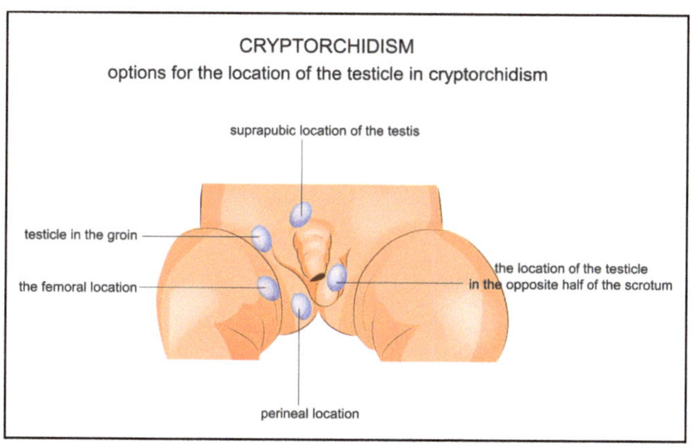

Phimosis: Can't retract foreskin over glans penis

Sx:

PE:

Dx:

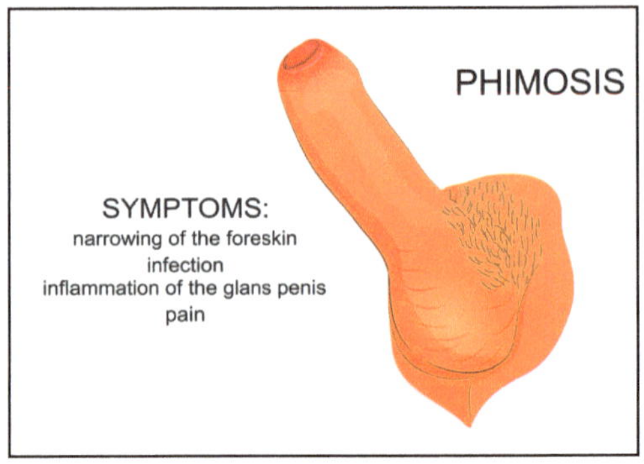

____

____

____

Tx:

Paraphimosis: Can't return foreskin EMERGENCY!

Sx:

PE:

Dx:

____

____

____

Tx:

Priapism:

Sx: Erection for > 2-4 hours without sexual excitement

PE:

Dx:

____

____

____

Tx:

Erectile Dysfunction:

Sx: Difficulty obtaining and/or maintaining an erection

PE:

Dx:

Tx:

Peyronie's Disease: Fibrosis of the tunica albuginea

Sx:

PE:

Dx: History & physical

Tx:

Epispadias:

Sx:

PE:

Dx:

Tx:

Hypospadias: **Urethral opening on posterior penis**

Sx:

PE:

Dx:

Tx:

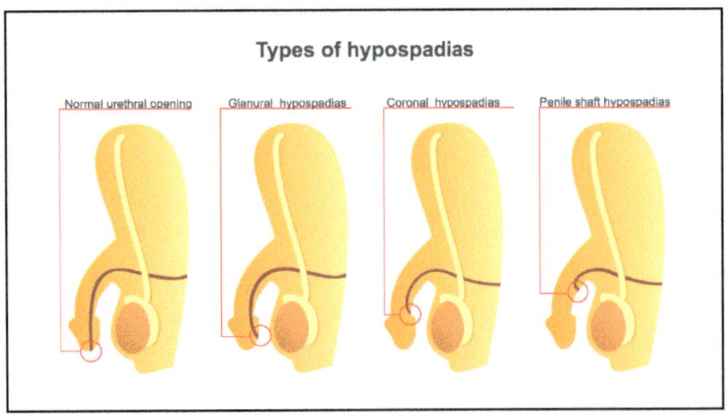

Benign Prostatic Hyperplasia (BPH):

Sx:

PE:

Dx:

Tx:

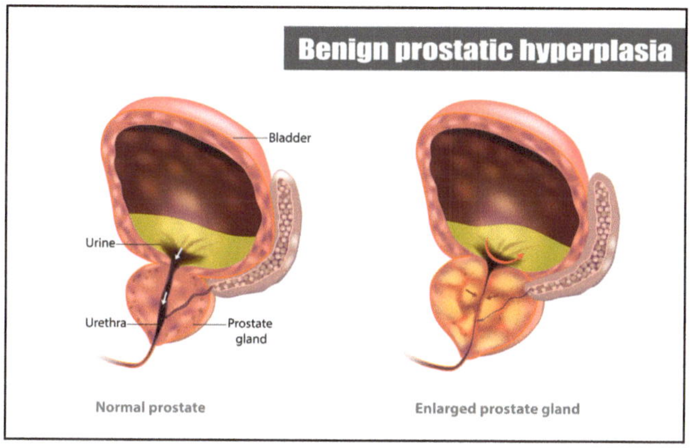

Diuretics: In Cardio

Medications

____________________: MOA = ____

Indication(s)=____

Side Effects = ____

Types/ Examples = ____

____

____

____________________: MOA = ____

Indication(s)=____

Side Effects = ____

Types/ Examples = ____

____

____

____________________: MOA = ____

Indication(s)=____

Side Effects = ____

Types/ Examples = ____

____

____

____________________: MOA = ____

Indication(s)=____

Side Effects = ____

Types/ Examples = ____

____

____

____________________: MOA = ____

Indication(s)=____

Side Effects = ____

Types/ Examples = ____

____

____

Medications

______________: MOA = ____________________

Indication(s)=____________________

Side Effects = ____________________

Types/ Examples = ____________________

____

____

______________: MOA = ____________________

Indication(s)=____________________

Side Effects = ____________________

Types/ Examples = ____________________

____

____

______________: MOA = ____________________

Indication(s)=____________________

Side Effects = ____________________

Types/ Examples = ____________________

____

____

______________: MOA = ____________________

Indication(s)=____________________

Side Effects = ____________________

Types/ Examples = ____________________

____

____

______________: MOA = ____________________

Indication(s)=____________________

Side Effects = ____________________

Types/ Examples = ____________________

____

____

Pediatrics

Milestones

2 months
Closure of posterior fontanelle

4 months
Colic resolves

6 months
Eyes should move in parallel without deviation and be consistently well-aligned

9 months

12 months

15 months
Walks alone

18 months

2 years
Puts 3 words together, feeds oneself, builds a tower with 7 cubes

3 years
Hearing deficit screening (pure tone audiometry)
Annual blood pressures should start at age 3

Reflexes

Moro (Startle)

Asymmetric Tonic Neck Reflex

Palmar Grasp

Rooting

Parachute

Immunization Schedule

Reasons to Delay Immunizations:

Pediatric Cardiology

Newborn Hypertrophic Cardiomyopathy:

Most common cause: Mutations in the genes for sarcomere proteins

Sx:

PE:

Dx:

____

____

____

Tx:

Pediatric Pulmonology

Respiratory Distress Syndrome: Type 2 pneumocytes fail to secrete surfactant

Sx: Tachycardia, nasal flaring, retractions, cyanosis

PE:

Dx:

____

____

____

Tx:

Pediatric Gastrointestinal

Meckel's Diverticulum: **Most common congenital GI tract anomaly**

Sx:

PE: "Currant jelly" stool

Dx: Meckel radionuclide scan or technetium scan

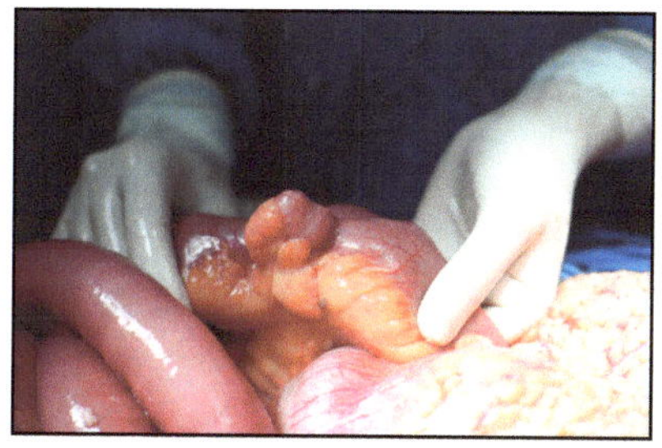

Tx:

Rule of 2's

- 2 years old
- 2 ft from ileocecal valve
- 2" long
- 2% of population

Constipation:

Sx: Frequency of stooling depends on age

PE:

Dx:

Tx:

Duodenal Atresia:

Sx:

PE: Bilious vomiting or mild form with distended abdomen

Dx: X-ray with "double bubble"

Tx:

Hirschsprung Disease: **Absence of ganglion cells in colon**

Sx: Failure to thrive, chronic constipation

PE: Abdominal distention

Dx:

Tx:

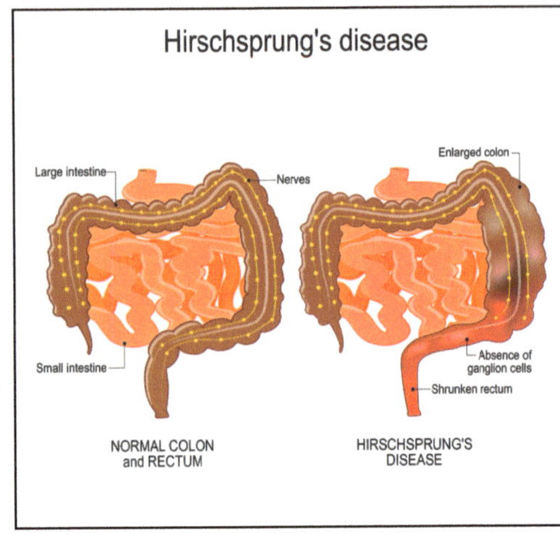

Neonatal Jaundice:

Sx: Yellowing of skin and conjunctiva

PE:

Dx:

Tx:

Pediatric Musculoskeletal

Osteogenesis Imperfecta:

Sx:

PE: Mild form - blue sclera, history of recurrent fractures, presenile deafness

Dx:

Tx:

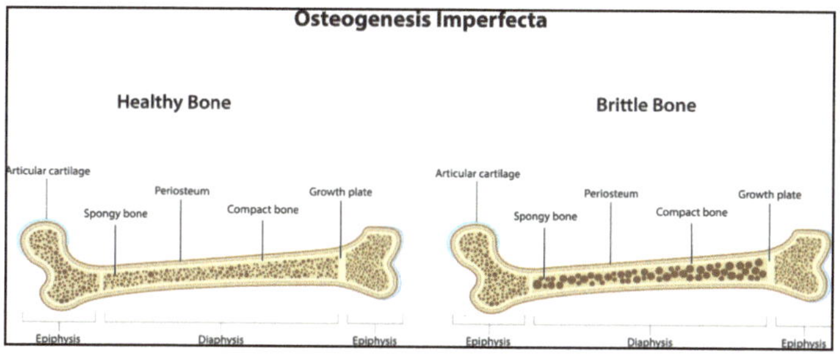

Duchenne Muscular Dystrophy:
Genetic defect on the short arm of the X chromosome. Usually males, diagnosed when toddlers

Sx:

PE:

Dx: CK, genetic analysis

Tx:

Osgood-Schlatter Disease:
Tibial Tuberosity Avulsion

Sx:

PE:

Dx: Clinical, X-ray

Tx:

Developmental Dysplasia/Hip Dysplasia:

Sx:

PE: < 3 months + Ortolani/Barlow maneuvers, > 3months + Galeazzi and Klisic test

Dx:

Tx:

Torticollis: Twisted neck, usually observed by 2-4 weeks of age

Sx: Head tilted to one side with chin pointed to other side

PE:

Dx:

Tx: Physical therapy

Slipped Capital Femoral Epiphysis:

Sx: Hip pain, external rotation/shortening of leg, limp

PE:

Dx: X-ray

Tx:

Marfan Syndrome:

Sx: Skeletal abnormalities (tall, joint laxity, pectus deformity), heart/skin/eye abnormalities

PE: + Thumb & wrist sign

Dx:

Tx:

Ehlers-Danlos Syndrome:

Sx: Joint hypermobility, skin hyperextensibility

PE:

Dx:

Tx:

Nursemaid's Elbow: **Radial head subluxation**

Sx:

PE: Holds affected arm close to body with elbow fully extended or slightly flexed and forearm pronated

Dx: History (pull injury), clinical, X-ray

Tx:

Pediatric EENT

Retinoblastoma:

Sx:

PE: Leukoria (abnormal red-light reflex)

Dx:

____ **Tx:**

____

____

Ophthalmia Neonatorum: **Eye infection within first 30 days of life**

Sx: Purulent conjunctivitis, swelling & exudate of eyelids

PE:

Dx:

____ **Tx:**

____

____

Pediatric Dermatology

Nevus Simplex (Macular Stain): "Stork Bite"

Sx: Pink/red patches usually on eyelids, glabella, or neck

PE:

Dx:

Tx:

Congenital Dermal Melanocytosis: "Mongolian Spots"

Sx: Blue/grey patches with unclear borders, usually in sacral and gluteal areas

PE:

Dx:

Tx:

Nevus Flammeus: "Port Wine Stains" (capillary malformations)

Sx: Pink/red, flat, blanchable lesions that respect midline, often on face

PE:

Dx:

Tx:

Café-au-lait Macules: Multiple lesions. Can be a sign of a systemic disorder

Sx: Flat pigmented lesions, usually a few shades darker than skin

PE:

Dx:

Tx:

Pediatric Endocrinology

Congenital Hypothyroidism:

Sx: Gradual, 3–6-month of age, poor appetite

PE: Enlarged abdomen & umbilical hernia, enlarged tongue, not meeting milestones

Dx:

____

____

____

Tx:

Chromosomal Abnormalities

Klinefelter Syndrome: Extra X chromosome

Sx:

PE: Gynecomastia, tall, thin, wide arm span, small phallus, & small, soft testis

Dx:

____

____

____

Tx:

Noonan Syndrome:

Sx:

PE: Short stature, webbed neck, pectus excavatum

Dx:

____

____

____

Tx:

21-Hydroxylase Deficiency: Congenital adrenal hyperplasia

Sx:

PE:

Dx: Early morning 17-hydroxyprogesterone level

____

____

____

Tx:

Fragile-X Syndrome:

Sx:

PE: Long face, protruding ears, male sex (usually), macroorchidism, macrocephaly, large jaw, frontal bossing

Dx:

Tx:

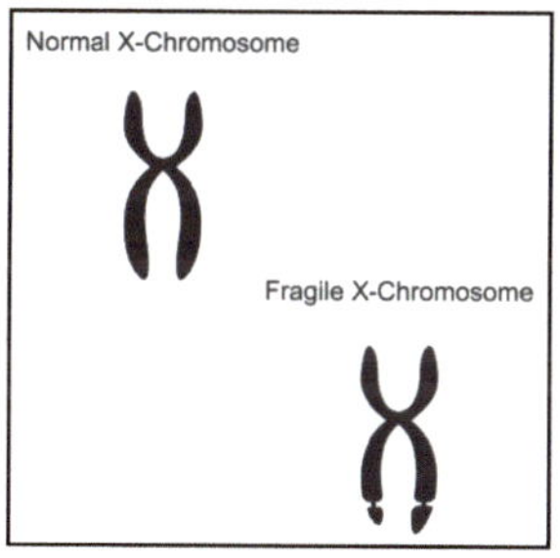

Down Syndrome: Trisomy 21

Sx:

PE:

Dx: Usually made through prenatal screening, usually clinical after birth, karyotype

Tx:

Prader-Willi Syndrome:

Sx: Large appetite, obesity, decreased cognition, hypogonadism

PE:

Dx: Genetic testing

Tx:

Pediatric Neurology

Niemann-Pick Disease: 2-6 months with progressive neurodegeneration, hypotonia, feeding difficulties

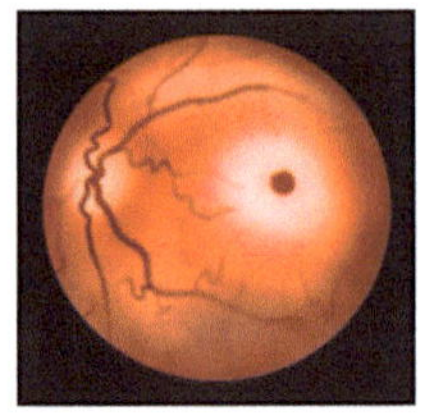

Sx:

PE: "Cherry red spot" on macula

Dx:

Tx:

Tay-Sachs Disease:

Sx:

PE: Hyperreflexia

Dx:

Tx:

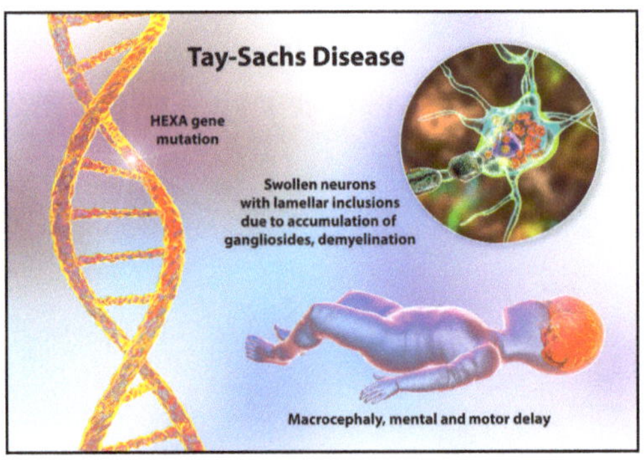

Rett Syndrome: Neurodegenerative disorder of unknown cause

Sx: Almost exclusively in females

PE:

Dx: DNA analysis of MECP2, FOX61, CDKL5

Tx:

Neurocysticercosis: Tapeworm infection

Sx:

PE:

Dx: CT and MRI

Tx:

Kernicterus: Brain damage from high bilirubin, develops within 1 year of birth

Sx: Cerebral palsy, sensorineural hearing loss, gaze abnormality, dental enamel hypoplasia

PE:

Dx:

Tx:

Reye Syndrome:

Sx: Lethargy, drowsiness, vomiting

PE: Hyperreflexia, Babinski sign, may have hepatomegaly

Dx:

____

____

____

Tx:

Spina Bifida:

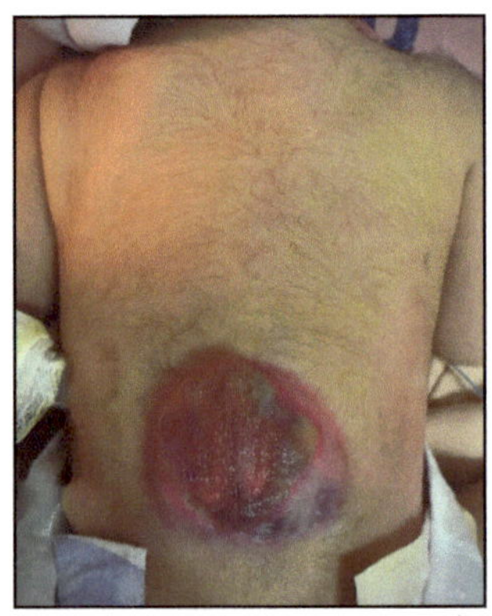

Sx:

PE:

Dx: CT or MRI is definitive test

Alpha-fetoprotein measured at 16-18 weeks in pregnancy

____

____

____

Tx:

Infantile Spasms:

Sx: Mixed flexor/extensor spasms, sudden flexion of neck, trunk, arms

PE:

Dx: Electroencephalogram (EEG)

______________________________ Tx:

____

____

Neuroblastoma:

Sx:

PE:

Dx: CBC, CMP, urine, or serum catecholamine metabolite levels

Refer to pediatric oncology/surgery for biopsy

______________________________ Tx:

____

____

Pediatric Hematology

Iron Poisoning:

Sx: Initial = vomiting and bloody diarrhea

Causes localized necrosis & hemorrhage

PE:

Dx:

Tx:

Fanconi Anemia: Autosomal recessive

Sx: Short stature, limb abnormalities

PE:

Dx: Labs = macrocytic, pancytopenia

Tx:

Increased risk for AML

Homocystinuria: **Disorder of amino acid metabolism**

Sx: Developmental delay, osteoporosis, thromboembolism, marfanoid appearance

PE:

Dx:

Tx:

Cephalohematoma: **Collection of blood between the skull & periosteum - does not cross suture lines**

Sx: Swelling of scalp that doesn't cross suture lines

PE:

Dx:

Tx:

Maternal Substance Use in Utero (Neonatal Abstinence Syndrome)

Cocaine Withdrawal:

Sx: Irritable, tremulous & inconsolable

PE: Increased pulse, small for gestational age, microcephaly, seizures

Dx:

____

____

____

Tx:

Alcohol: Fetal Alcohol Syndrome

Sx: Thin vermillion border, smooth philtrum, growth retardation, cognitive impairment, hyperactivity

PE:

Dx:

____

____

____

Tx:

Barbiturates:

Sx:

PE: Dysmorphic features (short nose & low nasal bridge), limb abnormalities

Dx:

____

____

____

Tx:

Opiate:

Sx: Placenta abruption, preterm labor, fetal growth restrictions, tremors

PE:

Dx:

Tx:

Heroin:

Sx: Irritable, not feeding or sleeping well, vomiting, loose stools, diaphoretic & high-pitched cry

PE: Fetal growth restrictions

Dx:

Tx:

Legg-Calve-Perthes Disease: In MSK

Kawasaki Syndrome: In MSK

Medications

______________: MOA = ______________

Indication(s)=______________

Side Effects = ______________

Types/ Examples = ______________

____

____

______________: MOA = ______________

Indication(s)=______________

Side Effects = ______________

Types/ Examples = ______________

____

____

______________: MOA = ______________

Indication(s)=______________

Side Effects = ______________

Types/ Examples = ______________

____

____

______________: MOA = ______________

Indication(s)=______________

Side Effects = ______________

Types/ Examples = ______________

____

____

______________: MOA = ______________

Indication(s)=______________

Side Effects = ______________

Types/ Examples = ______________

____

____

Medications

____________________: MOA = ____________________

Indication(s)=____________________

Side Effects = ____________________

Types/ Examples = ____________________

____

____

____________________: MOA = ____________________

Indication(s)=____________________

Side Effects = ____________________

Types/ Examples = ____________________

____

____

____________________: MOA = ____________________

Indication(s)=____________________

Side Effects = ____________________

Types/ Examples = ____________________

____

____

____________________: MOA = ____________________

Indication(s)=____________________

Side Effects = ____________________

Types/ Examples = ____________________

____

____

____________________: MOA = ____________________

Indication(s)=____________________

Side Effects = ____________________

Types/ Examples = ____________________

____

____

Appendix

Dermatology 268

Bibliography

Images:

iStock. "Royalty-Free Stock Images, Photos and Pictures." iStock, 2021, https://www.istockphoto.com/.

Shutterstock. "Royalty-Free Stock Images, Photos, Vectors, Video, and Music." Shutterstock, 2021, https://www.shutterstock.com/.

Resources:

Epocrates. "Point of Care Medical Applications." Epocrates, 2021, https://www.epocrates.com/.

Wolters Kluwer. "Solutions for Professionals." Wolters Kluwer, 2021, https://www.wolterskluwer.com/.

Williams, Dwayne A,. *PANCE Prep Pearls V3.* Independently published (November 28, 2019)

National Commission on Certification of Physician Assistants. "PANCE Blueprint." NCCPA, 2021, https://www.nccpa.net/become-certified/pance-blueprint/.

The Diagnostic and Statistical Manual of Mental Disorders version 5

www.ingramcontent.com/pod-product-compliance
Lightning Source LLC
Chambersburg PA
CBHW041320210926
51847CB00002B/8
9781971310060